The
Science
of
Beauty

The
Science
of
Beauty

DR MICHELLE WONG
aka Lab Muffin Beauty Science

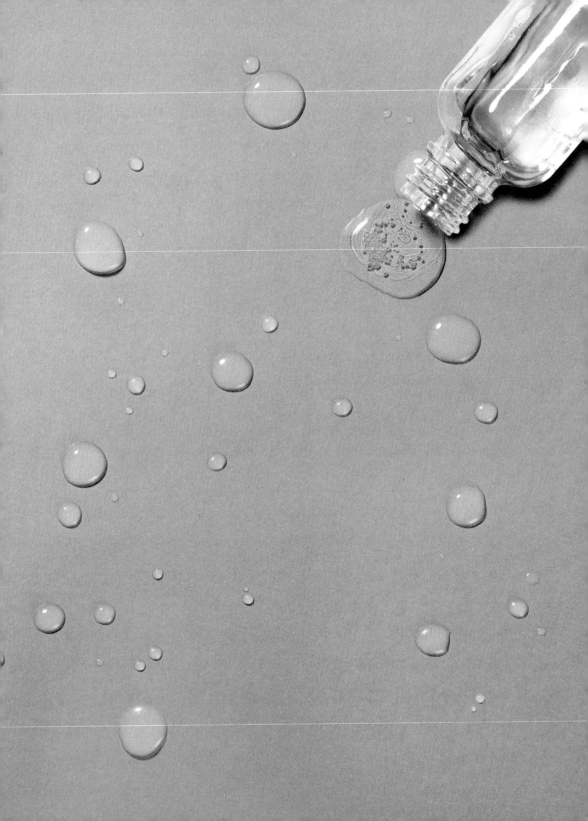

CONTENTS

What is beauty?

Subjective, valuable, and almost impossible to define, the concept of beauty is an inescapable part of how we experience the world – and one another.

As the saying goes, "Beauty is in the eye of the beholder." But many aesthetic preferences transcend boundaries: research has shown that certain facial traits, such as youth, symmetry, and happy-looking features, are universally regarded as attractive. One theory for this suggests that beauty may be an evolutionary instinct. A symmetrical face may imply health, while youth would suggest fertility. Another study created "average" faces by blending photos of people from the same country, then showed those images to people from that country. The more faces they blended together, the more attractive the face was deemed to be. In other words, each country (or culture) saw beauty in the faces that looked the most familiar to them.

At the same time, what is considered beautiful can vary from person to person, influenced by cultural norms, media representations, and individual tastes. Fashions can change from one year to the next, while different subcultures and groups have their own beauty and styling preferences. In some cultures, tanned skin is considered desirable; in others, paler skin is prized. Of course, it is difficult to disentangle modern beauty standards from the effects of colonization and globalization, which have spread Eurocentric beauty ideals. Together, these influences have led to the perpetuation of harmful standards in many societies. The pressure to conform can be immense, particularly for people whose looks are further from these often unrealistic ideals, amplifying body dissatisfaction and appearance-based discrimination.

The beauty industry

Beauty isn't just an abstract idea. It is big business, and beauty products and practices play many roles in our lives. Many have health or hygiene purposes, and even purely aesthetic functions are important: they allow self-expression, give us agency over

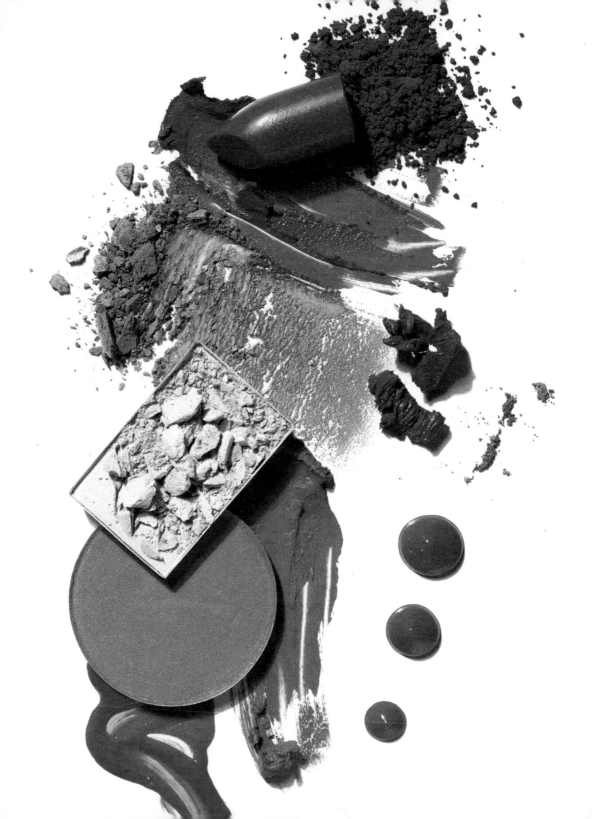

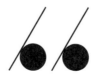

Beauty isn't just an abstract idea. It is big business, and beauty products and practices play many roles in our lives.

how we present ourselves to the world, and can boost our well-being and confidence. They can even have a financial function. Though unfair, studies have found that physically attractive people receive higher incomes on average, but makeup can be a way to level the playing field.

Yet the beauty industry has played a large role in perpetuating harmful beauty standards. For decades, airbrushed advertisements have reinforced narrow concepts of beauty, although in recent years there have been genuine attempts at diversity. Product marketing often exploits our insecurities, promising to make us look younger and thinner, and erase natural biological features like pores and cellulite. And there's a lot of money to be made from inventing problems for new products to solve. While this book will discuss the science behind common appearance-related concerns and how to address these, it's important to remember that these wants are often shaped by artificial expectations, and our looks do not dictate our value as people.

Myths and misinformation

I started Lab Muffin Beauty Science in 2011 because I was frustrated at the lack of accessible information on how beauty products worked, and the sheer volume of unrefuted misinformation online. Despite being a chemistry PhD student at the time, it was still incredibly challenging to unravel the science, so I wanted to make this information easily available to anyone interested. And clearly, many people were – my blog expanded onto Instagram, and then a YouTube channel as well.

But despite talking about beauty science for over a decade, there's no end of myths to debunk, and concepts to decipher. The beauty industry has traditionally been hesitant to reveal the scientific intricacies behind their products, leaving a vacuum for misinformation to grow. Many companies also profit from selling false hope and encouraging convenient misconceptions.

This book answers many of the questions I've been asked over the years, in a detailed but digestible way. It explains the science behind skincare, haircare, makeup, and nails, as well as beauty products themselves. I hope you'll find it fascinating, and empowering – it'll equip you with the knowledge to sort out fact from fiction when it comes to marketing claims, and work out which products will actually deliver the results you want.

Beauty basics

Are beauty products safe?

It's a common misconception that beauty products are largely unregulated, and that many mass market products are harmful to our health.

While there have been dangerous beauty products throughout history – heavy metals in 18th-century makeup, radioactive creams in the 1930s – the science surrounding health risks has progressed immensely, along with legal principles of liability. In most well-regulated marketplaces like the US and the EU, companies are legally responsible for demonstrating the safety of their products, and it is illegal to sell harmful products.

The safety of cosmetic ingredients is assessed by scientists using the same principles of toxicology used for evaluating foods and medications.

Cosmetic companies have a commercial interest in ensuring safe products. There is no financial benefit in hurting customers they've already convinced to buy their products, and negligence can lead to extensive litigation. Product recalls and safety infringement notices generate negative publicity and lead to large drops in sales. Standard practices have been developed within the industry to ensure that beauty products are safe before launch.

Ingredient selection

The safety of cosmetic ingredients is assessed by scientists, using the same principles of toxicology used for evaluating foods and medications. Safety assessments are published by independent expert bodies, including the Scientific Committee on Consumer Safety in the EU, the Cosmetics Ingredient Review in the US, and the Research Institute for Fragrance Materials.

The amount of the ingredient is particularly important, hence the saying "The dose makes the poison". If more ingredient molecules are present, they are more likely to interact with the body in a harmful (or beneficial) way. If the amount is extremely small, the likelihood of any molecules even reaching the relevant part of the body becomes infinitesimally small. This is why traces of heavy metals in beauty products usually aren't a big concern – modern scientific instruments can detect

RISK = HAZARD × EXPOSURE
To work out safety, scientists refer to risk, which
depends on both hazard and exposure.

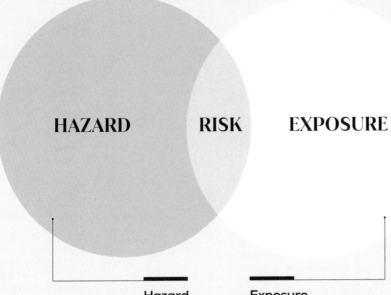

Hazard

The harms an ingredient might
potentially cause. Includes short-term
irritation and allergic reactions, as well
as longer-term effects like cancer and
endocrine disruption. Hazard
assessments consider:

- Tests on chemicals, cells, or isolated
  tissues (in vitro, ex vivo)
- Tests on animals (in vivo)
- Information from computer models
  (in silico)
- Clinical studies in human volunteers
- Epidemiological studies that look at
  population-level effects
- Case reports of people being
  harmed by the ingredient
- Data on similar ingredients that can
  be extrapolated (read-across)

Exposure

How consumers might be exposed
to the ingredient, which can involve:

- How much of the ingredient is
  used (dose)
- The ingredient's properties (e.g. how
  much is absorbed through skin)
- How it's used in products (wash-off
  or leave-on, frequency of use, how
  much is applied and where)
- The total exposure if the ingredient
  is in multiple products someone
  might use, including food and
  household products
- Foreseeable misuse

minute amounts of substances, well below the threshold for harm. Since risk depends on both hazard and exposure, a highly hazardous ingredient can still be used safely. For example, botulinum toxin (botox) is the most toxic substance known, but depending on exposure it can be very safe (if a tiny amount is injected in a face muscle by a trained professional) or very dangerous (large amounts eaten in contaminated food, causing botulism).

From hazard and exposure data, toxicologists can calculate the concentrations of ingredients that can be safely used in different products. Cosmetic formulators refer to their recommendations when creating products. Concentration limits established by regulatory agencies are sometimes written into law.

Margin of safety

A large margin of safety is built into these recommendations. This means that the amounts used are a tiny fraction (usually $1/100$) of a dose that would still not be harmful, based on current scientific evidence.

PRODUCT SAFETY

BEFORE LAUNCH

Stability testing
Product is stored under different conditions to make sure it doesn't change too much over time. Heat is used to simulate longer storage at room temperature. Colour, smell, pH, and texture are recorded.

Processes are conducted by trained personnel following documented protocols to minimize mix-ups and contamination.

Monitoring can quickly identify issues.

POST-MARKET SURVEILLANCE (COSMETOVIGILANCE)

Unexpected side effects are reported by consumers and doctors, and monitored by both regulators and cosmetic companies. Regulators also occasionally analyse products on the market. Faulty or unsafe products may be recalled.

Preservative efficacy testing
An effective preservative system is needed to prevent microbial overgrowth, which can cause irritation, infections, and even injury. During testing, microbes are added to products and their growth is measured.

Safety testing
Irritancy and allergenicity are tested by applying products to volunteers. Both worst-case and real-use scenarios are tested. Tests on live animals were used in the past, but these have been almost completely replaced by other methods.

MANUFACTURING

Facilities, equipment, and packaging are carefully cleaned, and tested for contamination.

Raw ingredients are analysed before use (e.g. microbes, impurities).

While not legally required in many countries, most cosmetics are produced under good manufacturing practices (GMP), to ensure consistent quality and prevent contamination.

SAFETY TIPS

The vast majority of beauty products are very safe, but following a few guidelines will ensure extra protection against harm.

Buy from reputable stores and brands to avoid products that may not follow standard safety practices (e.g. counterfeit products).

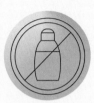

Do not use recalled products.

Follow directions for use, including storage instructions, expiry dates, and any occupational safety requirements.

If you have a concerning reaction to a product, seek medical attention.

Are natural beauty products better or safer?

Natural products and ingredients are often marketed as being safer. But this claim is misleading for many reasons.

Natural isn't well-defined

No one can agree on exactly what counts as "natural". Everything technically originated on Earth, so in a sense all ingredients are natural. But to get into a jar of cream safely, ingredients need to undergo extensive processing, so they're all also quite unnatural by the time they reach us.

Additionally, any substance found in nature can be theoretically made in a laboratory, and the natural and synthetic versions will have identical impacts on your body – their molecules will be exactly the same.

Many ingredients originally sourced from nature are made synthetically for cosmetic use. This can have many advantages:
- Reduces strain on natural resources
- Often lower cost
- More predictable composition and properties (such as any contaminants present)

Some certification bodies have definitions for "natural" or "naturally derived", but there is much disagreement between standards, and the distinctions drawn are quite arbitrary. For example, petroleum jelly is usually considered "unnatural", even though it's a purified extract of natural crude oil – impurities are removed, but the petroleum jelly molecules are unchanged from when they were extracted from the ground.

Natural isn't automatically safer

It's a myth that natural substances are inherently safer. Many dangerous contaminants in beauty products throughout history were natural, including lead, asbestos, and mould.

Natural ingredients can be riskier than synthetic alternatives. For example, natural fragrance materials often contain common allergens, but they can be avoided when creating synthetic blends. Synthetic iron oxide pigments are almost always used in makeup, because natural iron oxides are often contaminated with toxic heavy metals.

Synthetic ingredients can be produced in a more consistent way, so their properties and effects are far more predictable.

Natural ingredients aren't more effective

Nature has provided us with many valuable substances, including medications. But evolution is geared towards having organisms survive long enough to reproduce. There's no evolutionary pressure for a plant to produce substances that benefit humans, so it's largely luck when a natural ingredient happens to be helpful.

On the other hand, synthetic molecules can be customized to improve their properties. There's also a lot of variation in natural products, which raises quality control issues. A single plant extract can contain thousands of unique chemicals, so its exact composition and subsequent effects depend on many factors like climate, season, and extraction method. In contrast, synthetic ingredients can be produced in a more consistent way, so their properties and effects are far more predictable.

The bottom line: an ingredient's origin doesn't say much about its safety or effectiveness. Every ingredient needs to be evaluated on its own merits, whether natural or synthetic.

NATURAL VS SYNTHETIC INGREDIENTS

Synthetic ingredients are often inspired by naturally occurring substances, with modifications that improve their properties.

Double bonds are removed from squalene to make squalane, which improves its stability.

Squalene (natural)
Found in shark liver oil, olive oil, and human sebum.

Squalane (synthetic)
Synthesized from sugarcane via microbiological and chemical processes.

Squalane is more stable than squalene, while having similar moisturizing properties.

Are cosmetic ingredients dangerous?

"Free from" lists are common in beauty marketing. However, the vast majority of the ingredients mentioned have not been linked to health issues when used in the context of cosmetics.

Often these fears come from cell or animal studies that used much higher amounts than we'd get from beauty products, frequently millions of times higher. Sometimes it's from reports of weak links, or outlier findings that cannot be reproduced. Many ingredients have been removed from products due to sensationalist media coverage and unscrupulous marketing, rather than any legitimate safety issue. The replacement ingredients are usually less studied, and may have greater health risks.

”

Many ingredients have been removed from products due to sensationalist media coverage and unscrupulous marketing.

Safety assessors regularly recommend reducing the use of older ingredients, but this is part of a gradual process of minimizing even small risks, as new science emerges and alternatives are developed. These changes are almost always because of small effects in animals, or changes in biochemical measurements that may or may not be linked to health problems – it's incredibly rare that anyone has actually been harmed.

Parabens

"Free from parabens" is one of the most popular claims. Parabens are a diverse family of preservatives that have been used widely in cosmetics and food for about a century, due to their safety, low allergenicity, and effectiveness.

Much of the concern is around their oestrogenic activity and potential endocrine disruption, but studies have repeatedly found that parabens are thousands to millions of times weaker than natural oestrogen.

In 2004, a study reported that parabens were found in breast cancer tissue. However, the levels found were not compared to non-cancerous tissue, and some of the parabens seemed to have been introduced during the experiment. Nevertheless, this sparked a lot of media attention, and calls for parabens to be removed.

Many parabens (methyl-, ethyl-, propyl- and butylparaben) are still permitted in cosmetics in most regions, due to the large body of scientific evidence demonstrating their safety. Some larger parabens have been banned in the EU, not due to evidence of harm but lack of data, and their inherently higher (but still extremely low) oestrogenicity. In 2021, EU safety assessors found that using 17 products daily, all with the maximum allowed amount of propylparaben, would expose you to $^1/_{12,500}$ of an amount still considered safe.

Regrettable substitution

Since demonized ingredients usually have important uses, they need to be replaced with alternatives, which potentially increases health risks.

Many preservatives that replaced parabens are less effective, leading to some recalls of improperly preserved products, with visible microbial growth.

Relative risks of propylparaben
Recommended ingredient use levels have large margins of safety. Here we can see the propylparaben exposure from beauty products relative to levels still considered safe.

Key

Little to no health impact expected

Usual "safe" limit

Actual propylparaben exposure, if 17 products with maximum allowed concentration used daily

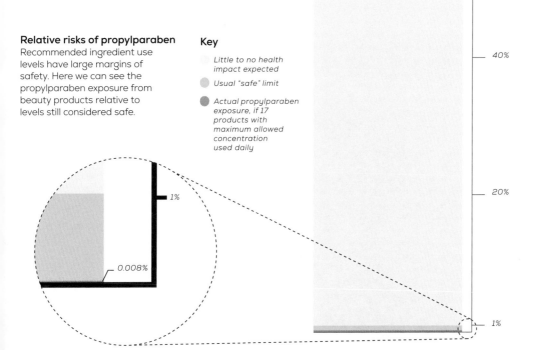

100%

80%

60%

40%

20%

1%

1%

0.008%

There is usually substantially less data on alternative preservatives, so they may not actually be safer. For example, increased use of methylisothiazolinone has led to an "epidemic" rise in allergic contact dermatitis. The American Contact Dermatitis Society named parabens the "non-allergen of the year" in 2019 to highlight their relative safety.

Other demonized ingredients

Fragrance is a closely guarded trade secret, so the generic term "fragrance" is often used on ingredient lists. This secrecy has led to many concerns about the safety of the individual components. However, 80% of the global volume of fragrance is produced by members of the International Fragrance Association (IFRA) and must follow their safety guidelines, which are based on toxicological principles of risk (see pp12–15). IFRA standards are independently reviewed by scientists without ties to the fragrance industry, and widely recognized by regulators. However, the secrecy surrounding fragrance can be a problem if you're allergic to specific fragrance ingredients, in which case it might be more practical to seek fragrance-free products. Some brands are beginning to disclose individual fragrance components online.

Phthalates are primarily used to make plastics more flexible. There are around ten phthalates commonly used in consumer products, each posing different health risks. Some phthalates are suspected endocrine disrupters, but cosmetics are not a large source of exposure to these.

Diethyl phthalate (DEP) is the only phthalate widely found in cosmetics due to a large amount of evidence confirming its safety. It's used as a solvent and denaturant in perfumes.

Dimethyl phthalate (DMP) and dibutyl phthalate (DBP) were historically used in hairspray and nail polish. Although the amounts in cosmetics were too low to cause harm, they were largely phased out by 2010 as a precaution.

Traces of other phthalates have been detected in cosmetics, likely due to leaching from plastic packaging. These levels are expected to have little to no effect, and would be insignificant compared to exposures from other sources like food packaging.

BEAUTY MYTHS

INGREDIENT SCANNING APPS

Many apps and websites claim to help you avoid toxic products by giving each product a simple score. They often list ingredient hazards with references to scientific studies, and can appear convincing.

However, these are rarely developed with cosmetic or toxicology experts. Scores are usually based purely on ingredient lists, without considering exposure and dose, which are both crucial for evaluating safety. The dangers listed are usually from cell and animal studies, and aren't directly relevant to normal product use – for example, ingredients are fed to animals or injected in most protocols.

NOT IN COSMETIC PRODUCTS

Butyl benzyl phthalate

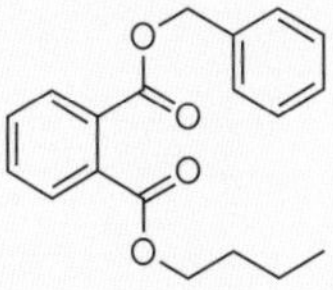

Diisobutyl phthalate

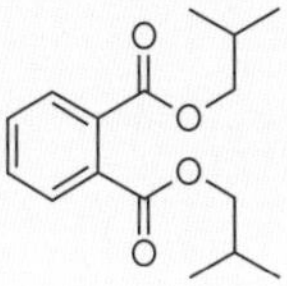

Diethylhexyl phthalate

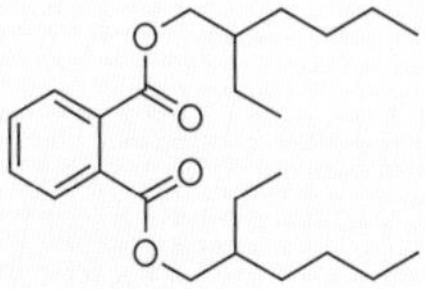

Phthalates in cosmetics

Many apps and websites warn about the risks of phthalates in cosmetics, based on data from phthalates NOT found in cosmetics. Only diethyl phthalate is commonly used in cosmetic products, due to its good safety profile.

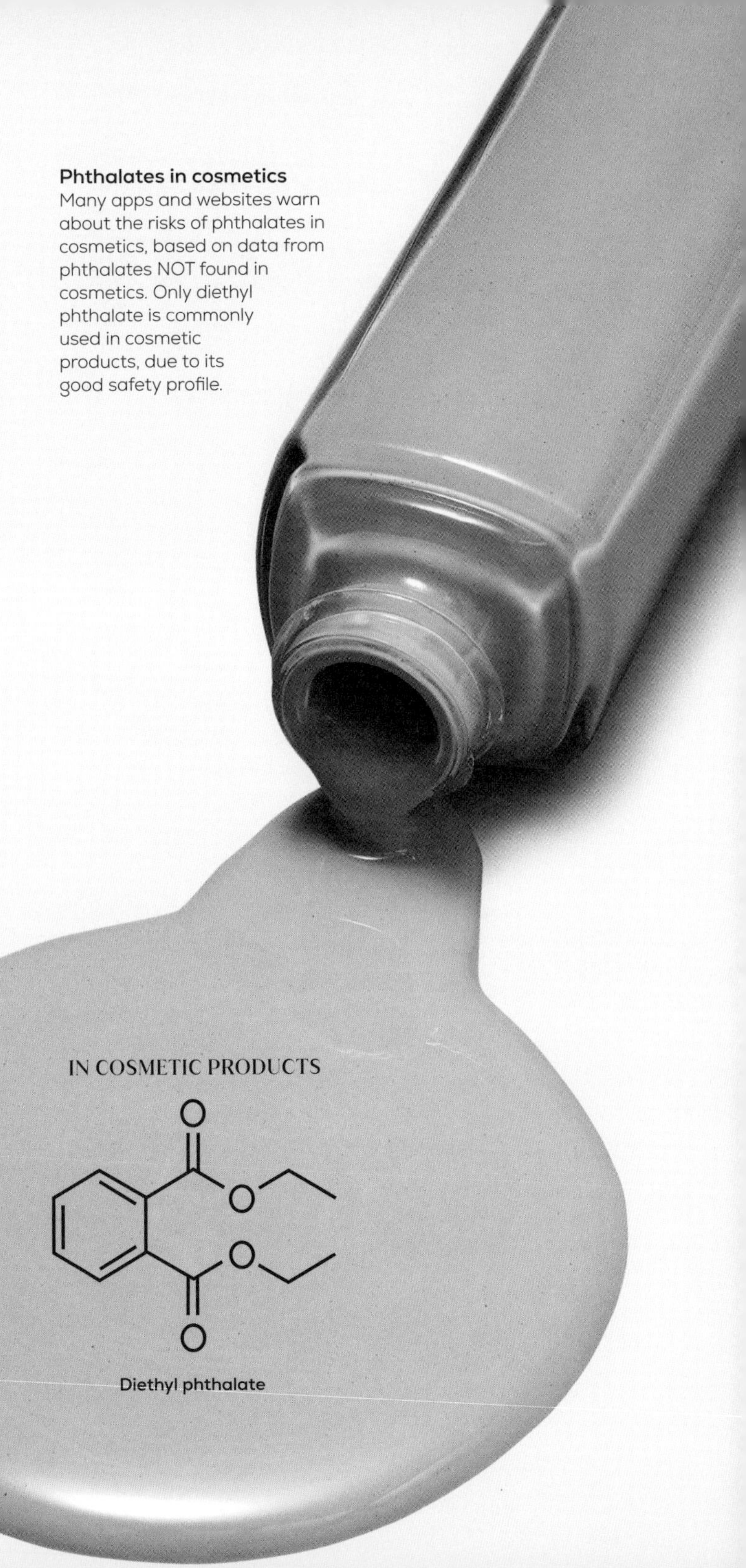

IN COSMETIC PRODUCTS

Diethyl phthalate

Are expensive products better?

The price of a beauty product doesn't tell us much about its quality or effectiveness.

Some factors that directly improve product performance can add to its cost, like rigorous product testing, formula optimization, higher-quality ingredients, and special delivery systems.

However, cost can also be driven up by factors unrelated to performance. Many effective ingredients are inexpensive, while call-out ingredients used more for marketing purposes than for established benefits can be costly, like organic botanical extracts or diamond. Fragrance is often one of the most expensive components of a product.

Then there's packaging. High-end products tend to have expensive features like embossing, and heavy luxury containers add to transport costs. However, higher-priced packaging can still be important, as it protects the product and can lengthen its shelf life.

Other overheads that can push prices up include marketing costs (e.g. advertising campaigns, celebrity endorsements), operational costs (e.g. warehousing, shipping, payment processing), retail stockist mark-ups, and seller commissions.

What's in a (brand) name?

Many variations between brands change the costs involved. Larger brands can benefit from economies of scale: upfront expenses, like formula development costs, are distributed over more units. This is why many supermarket products can be created with heavy research investment, despite their budget-friendly prices. Brands operating in different locations will have different costs for energy, labour, and transport.

Finally, cost can be determined simply by customer expectation. While retail prices are almost always above cost prices, the exact mark-up is usually based on competitor prices and consumer perception. For example, a luxury brand would never sell a cheap lipstick even if production costs decreased drastically, as it would communicate a lower brand value.

Call-out ingredients, like organic botanical extracts or diamond, can be costly.

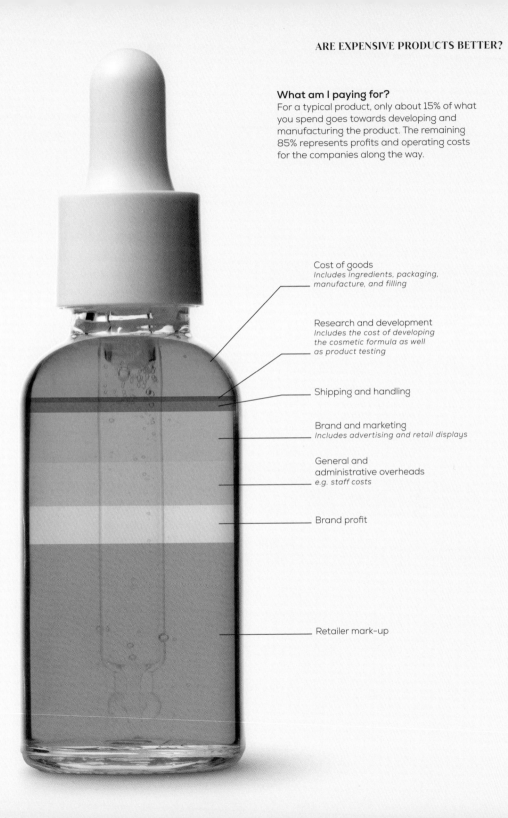

ARE EXPENSIVE PRODUCTS BETTER?

What am I paying for?
For a typical product, only about 15% of what you spend goes towards developing and manufacturing the product. The remaining 85% represents profits and operating costs for the companies along the way.

Cost of goods
Includes ingredients, packaging, manufacture, and filling

Research and development
Includes the cost of developing the cosmetic formula as well as product testing

Shipping and handling

Brand and marketing
Includes advertising and retail displays

General and administrative overheads
e.g. staff costs

Brand profit

Retailer mark-up

A luxury brand would never sell a cheap product even if production costs decreased drastically, as it would communicate a lower brand value.

What is an active ingredient?

Active or functional ingredients help a product fulfil its main function. The most potent components of a product, they drive its intended effects, from moisturizing to anti-aging.

UV filters
These protect against UV. They're the main functional ingredients in sunscreens, but are also added to other products to protect UV-sensitive ingredients.

Hair conditioning agents
These coat hair strands to make them smoother, shinier, and protect them against damage. They include cationic surfactants, silicones, and polymers.

Fixatives
Used in hair styling products to hold the shape of hair. They are also found in makeup fixing sprays, mascaras, and sunscreens to create more continuous films.

Skin conditioning or moisturizing agents
These help skin retain water, making it feel smoother and softer. They're found in many products, including moisturizing creams, body wash, and lipstick. There are three main categories: occlusives, emollients, and humectants (see pp60–61).

Abrasives
Solid grains that physically clean surfaces by scrubbing. They're found in scrubs and toothpastes.

Cleansing surfactants
Used in face cleansers, body washes, and shampoos to remove oily deposits from skin and hair.

COMMON SKINCARE ACTIVES

In skincare, the term "actives" usually refers to ingredients that are intended to produce a longer-lasting effect. However, the line between "active" and "inactive" is blurry, since skin responds to many environmental influences, including water.

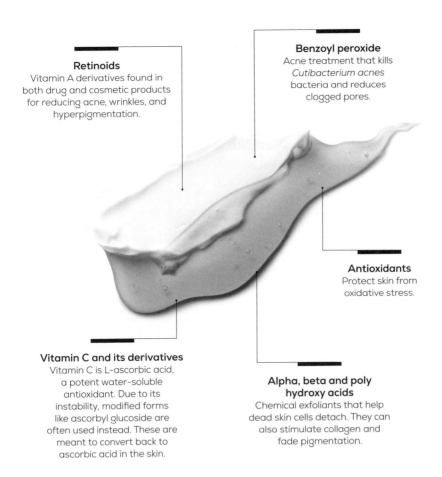

Retinoids
Vitamin A derivatives found in both drug and cosmetic products for reducing acne, wrinkles, and hyperpigmentation.

Benzoyl peroxide
Acne treatment that kills *Cutibacterium acnes* bacteria and reduces clogged pores.

Antioxidants
Protect skin from oxidative stress.

Vitamin C and its derivatives
Vitamin C is L-ascorbic acid, a potent water-soluble antioxidant. Due to its instability, modified forms like ascorbyl glucoside are often used instead. These are meant to convert back to ascorbic acid in the skin.

Alpha, beta and poly hydroxy acids
Chemical exfoliants that help dead skin cells detach. They can also stimulate collagen and fade pigmentation.

What do the different ingredients in beauty products do?

Active or functional ingredients are central to a product's main function. But the other ingredients have important roles too.

"Inactive" structural and supportive ingredients are essential to a product's texture, stability, and preservation. They can also enhance the efficacy of active ingredients and improve product safety.

Solvents

These dissolve other ingredients, or simply act as the bulk of the product to improve application. Solvents can also help ingredients absorb into skin or hair.

Viscosity modifiers

These adjust the thickness of a product, which changes how it spreads during use or dispenses from packaging. They can also help prevent product separation. Some viscosity modifiers prevent solid ingredients like pigments from settling. Viscosity modifiers are used in almost every product, so thicker products aren't necessarily more concentrated.

pH adjusters

Usually added near the end of the production process to change the pH (acidity) to the required level. For example, most skin products are adjusted to pH 4–6 to match the skin's natural acidity, while permanent hair dyes are adjusted to pH 9–11 to help them penetrate into the hair shaft.

Preservatives

These reduce bacterial and fungal growth in products to a safe level. Without an effective preservative system, products can spoil within days and cause irritation or infection. "Self-preserving" products are inherently hostile to microbes and don't need preservatives. This includes products with very low water content, high alcohol content, high acidity or alkalinity, or truly airtight packaging.

Antioxidants

These neutralize reactive free radicals that often form with oxygen exposure, preventing them from damaging other ingredients. For example, many plant oils become rancid through oxidation. Antioxidants can also reduce irritation from potentially harsh products, and protect skin and hair from oxidative stress.

Chelating agents

These stabilize formulas by trapping metal ions that may be introduced as impurities, as they can cause rancidity and colour changes, and compromise the preservative system. Chelating agents also help cleansers work better in hard water by trapping metal ions.

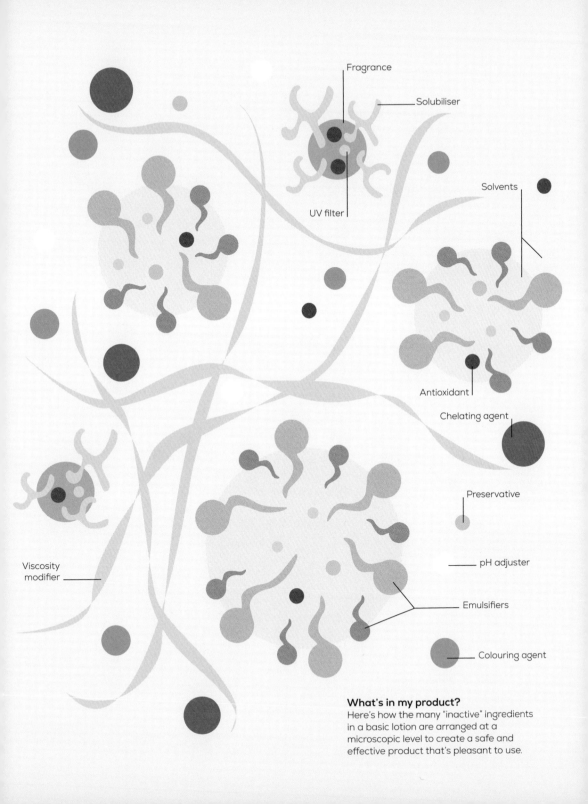

Fragrance

Solubiliser

UV filter

Solvents

Antioxidant

Chelating agent

Preservative

pH adjuster

Emulsifiers

Colouring agent

Viscosity modifier

What's in my product?
Here's how the many "inactive" ingredients in a basic lotion are arranged at a microscopic level to create a safe and effective product that's pleasant to use.

UV filters

These protect UV-sensitive ingredients such as fragrances and some skincare actives from degradation.

Emulsifiers

These are part of a wider class of ingredients called surfactants. Emulsifiers keep water- and oil-soluble components mixed together in an emulsion for many months or even years, without separating. Most beauty products are emulsions, including creams, lotions, liquid foundations, and hair conditioners (see diagram below).

Solubilisers

Like emulsifiers, these are a type of surfactant. They suspend very small droplets of oil-soluble ingredients like fragrances in water, while keeping the product transparent.

Fragrances

These add a pleasant scent, or hide the odours of raw ingredients. Fragrance strongly influences how consumers perceive other aspects of the product ("halo effect"). In one study, the same shampoo fragranced with citrus was judged to make hair silkier and smoother than when it had a camphor scent. Since fragrances are a closely guarded trade secret, they are often listed under the umbrella term "fragrance" or "parfum" in ingredient lists. Essential oils are commonly used for fragrance, but are often listed individually.

Colouring agents

In small quantities, these add colour to the product. They are included in products like makeup and hair dye in larger quantities, to add colour during application. Colouring agents include dyes (water-soluble) and pigments (insoluble, found as solid particles).

Flavouring agents

Used in lip and oral care products to mask unpleasant tastes of raw ingredients, or to add a distinctive flavour.

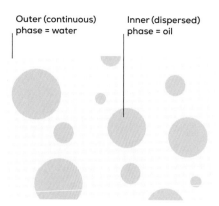

Oil-in-water emulsion (e.g. body lotion)
Droplets of oil dispersed in water.

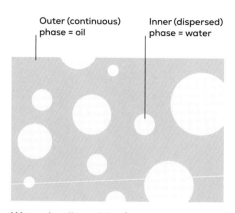

Water-in-oil emulsion (e.g. sunscreen)
Droplets of water dispersed in oil (often silicones).

Does packaging matter?

Beauty products are formulated with the packaging in mind, and tested in the final packaging. The choice of packaging depends on a number of factors.

Product stability

Packaging can protect ingredients that are light- and oxygen-sensitive. Opaque packaging limits light exposure, while oxygen can diffuse through some packaging materials but not others. Some products can also react with certain materials.

Usability

Certain product textures are suited to some packaging and not others. For example, thick products are difficult to squeeze from droppers, while thin products spill easily out of jars.

Marketing and consumer psychology

Colours, materials, and fonts are carefully chosen to optimize how consumers perceive the product, and to align with expectations. For example, luxury products usually come in heavier packaging, often made of glass.

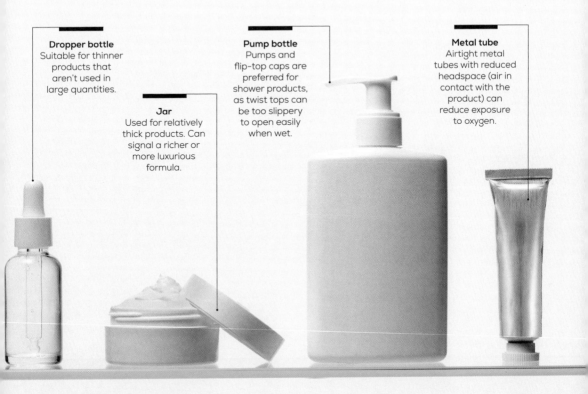

Dropper bottle
Suitable for thinner products that aren't used in large quantities.

Jar
Used for relatively thick products. Can signal a richer or more luxurious formula.

Pump bottle
Pumps and flip-top caps are preferred for shower products, as twist tops can be too slippery to open easily when wet.

Metal tube
Airtight metal tubes with reduced headspace (air in contact with the product) can reduce exposure to oxygen.

What do marketing buzzwords mean?

There are many buzzwords used in beauty marketing. However, most aren't regulated, so there aren't any guarantees about what exactly they mean.

"Hypoallergenic"
This suggests a product has been formulated to reduce the chance of allergic reactions. Ideally, the finished product would have been tested extensively on many sensitive-skinned people. However, many "hypoallergenic" products simply avoid using common allergens.

"Salon strength"
This marketing term, along with "clinical strength" or "professional strength", is meant to suggest a more powerful product than usual, but this isn't always the case. However, some products available for professional use in salons cannot be sold to consumers.

"Chemical-free"
This is a meaningless term – everything is made of chemicals.

"Cosmeceutical"
This term implies that a skincare product has longer-term "pharmaceutical" benefits on top of purely "cosmetic" appearance-based effects. Some countries like Japan and Korea have special categories of products in between cosmetics and drugs, but "cosmeceutical" is largely a marketing term used by products that are legally cosmetics. They can be less potent and less rigorously tested than some "non-cosmeceutical" products.

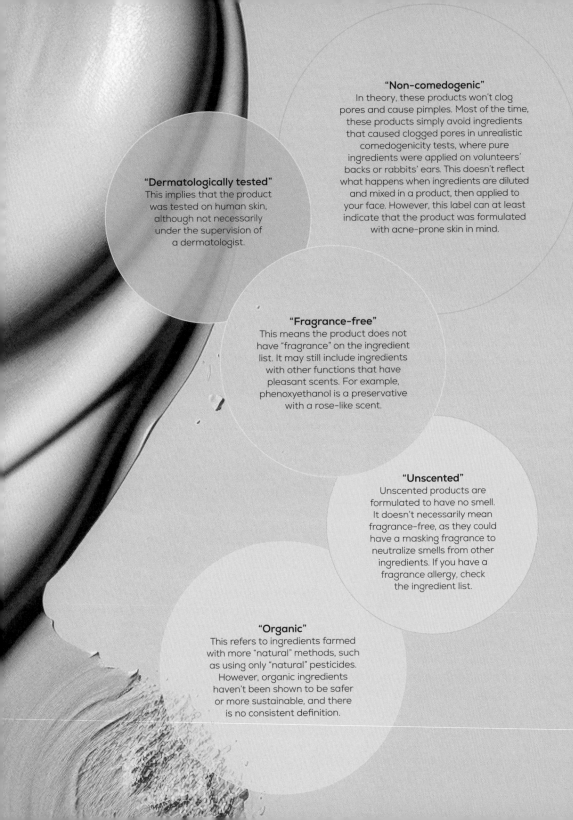

"Non-comedogenic"
In theory, these products won't clog pores and cause pimples. Most of the time, these products simply avoid ingredients that caused clogged pores in unrealistic comedogenicity tests, where pure ingredients were applied on volunteers' backs or rabbits' ears. This doesn't reflect what happens when ingredients are diluted and mixed in a product, then applied to your face. However, this label can at least indicate that the product was formulated with acne-prone skin in mind.

"Dermatologically tested"
This implies that the product was tested on human skin, although not necessarily under the supervision of a dermatologist.

"Fragrance-free"
This means the product does not have "fragrance" on the ingredient list. It may still include ingredients with other functions that have pleasant scents. For example, phenoxyethanol is a preservative with a rose-like scent.

"Unscented"
Unscented products are formulated to have no smell. It doesn't necessarily mean fragrance-free, as they could have a masking fragrance to neutralize smells from other ingredients. If you have a fragrance allergy, check the ingredient list.

"Organic"
This refers to ingredients farmed with more "natural" methods, such as using only "natural" pesticides. However, organic ingredients haven't been shown to be safer or more sustainable, and there is no consistent definition.

Can I trust the research in beauty marketing?

Under advertising laws, companies need to back up any product claims. But marketing claims often push the limits, to the point of being misleading!

Cosmetic claims vs drug claims

In most regions, cosmetic products can only legally make claims about changing the appearance of the body, not its structure or function – regardless of what the evidence shows. There are also limits on claims regarding diseases.

This is why many products use qualifiers in their claims. For example, a cream might claim to *"reduce the appearance of wrinkles"*, even if their tests show that it reduces wrinkles by boosting skin's collagen production.

However, another product might claim to *"reduce the appearance of wrinkles"* while only covering them up. And a product that says it *"reduces wrinkles by stimulating collagen production"* might sound more powerful – but this is usually an illegal drug claim, which reveals that the brand did not do their due diligence, and may have skipped other steps in their product development process.

Drug claims vs cosmetic claims
These are some examples of therapeutic claims that can be made only by drugs in many regions, and similar, weaker, cosmetic claims, which mostly concern appearance.

THERAPEUTIC (DRUG) CLAIMS

These therapeutic claims are usually only allowed for approved drugs, which meet legally recognized criteria for effectiveness, such as passing specific clinical tests.

"FADES PIGMENTATION"

"REDUCES CELLULITE"

"REDUCES WRINKLES"

NON-THERAPEUTIC (COSMETIC) CLAIMS

Cosmetics can typically only make claims about changes in appearance, and may use more indirect language to describe their effects.

"REDUCES APPEARANCE OF PIGMENTATION"

"SKIN LOOKS SMOOTHER"

"CONTAINS RETINOL"

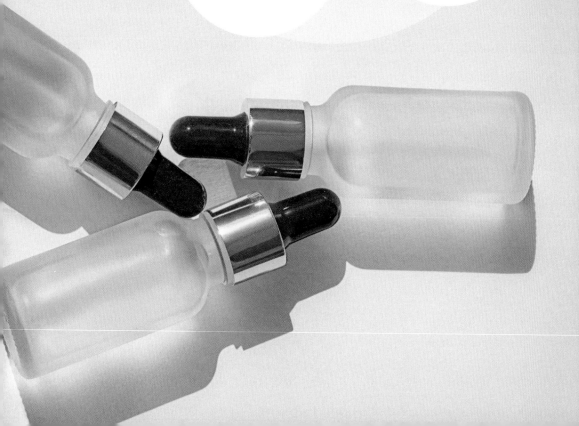

Product claims vs ingredient claims

Some claims are based on directly testing the product, while others are based on data about the ingredients it contains.

For example, "*95% of users noticed less hair breakage after eight weeks*" is based on how a specific product performed in a test, and will give a more accurate idea of its effectiveness. However, these tests cost more to run.

"*Contains [ingredient] that can increase skin hydration by 46% in three hours*" is an ingredient claim, based on how it performed in a different formula. This is a less reliable indication of a product's effectiveness, since the overall formulation makes a big difference. For example, the formula can increase ingredient penetration into skin, change how it distributes along hair strands, or protect ingredients from decomposition.

"Free-from" ingredient claims, which state what the product does not contain, are almost always based on misconceptions around ingredient safety, not actual risks (see p18).

Clinical, in vivo, ex vivo, in vitro tests

Many different tests are used to support product claims. For many claims, clinical (in vivo) tests are the most reliable. These involve testing the product on human volunteers under carefully controlled conditions, and its effects are measured objectively, like with an instrument. "*Reduces skin dryness by 55%*" is an example of a clinical testing claim. Clinical tests are usually used for SPF, skin hydration (using an instrument that measures conductivity), hair count, and irritation (human repeat insult patch tests).

Clinical claims will usually mention who the product was tested on and how

"Clinically proven" is not a regulated term, so it doesn't guarantee rigorous testing.

they used the product – for example, 80 white women aged 40–50 after eight weeks of daily use. In general, more test subjects will give more reliable results.

However, clinical tests are not always conducted fairly, and may not reflect actual use. This is sometimes to make the product look better, but it can also be necessary to make sure the test is fair. For example, many skincare serums are tested on their own. However, most consumers would be using it alongside their usual products, but if these were used in the test it could distort the results.

"Clinically proven" is not a regulated term, so it doesn't guarantee rigorous testing. Clinical testing is not always necessary. For example, hair is dead once it leaves the scalp, so conditioner performance is often evaluated using hair tresses. Some tests can be performed on detached samples of skin. Cell studies are also used to investigate how ingredients work. These are called "ex vivo" or "in vitro" tests.

Consumer perception tests

Claims like "*94% of users agreed that hair was stronger*" come from consumer perception tests, where users are asked for their opinion on how the product performed. These are subjective, but indicate how noticeable results will be. They are sometimes necessary to use, as objective measurements can be illegal drug claims. However, many external factors can influence someone's perception of how well a product worked, due to the halo effect. For example, in one experiment, a moisturizer was considered greasier when the fragrance was removed. The wording of questions can also change the results.

NAVIGATING PRODUCT CLAIMS

For the best chance of getting a product that works:
- Choose products with ingredients that can potentially act in the way you want, and have been shown to work in independent, peer-reviewed studies.
- Ideally, look for product claims from tests with objective measures and people similar to you.
- Try to find before-and-after photos with consistent lighting and minimal manipulation, and consumer perception claims to get an idea of what results to expect.
- Look for brands known to invest in research and development, e.g. they have scientists on staff and publish high-quality scientific studies.
- Read reviews from people with similar skin and hair to yours.
- Be wary of products with illegal claims.

What do beauty product labels tell us?

The information on the back of a product can guide you in making an informed choice.

Product labels can often seem confusing, so here's how to make sense of them.

What does an ingredient list tell us?

In most countries, ingredients in cosmetics must be listed on the packaging, according to specific rules. They can be extremely helpful if you need to check for ingredients you should avoid, like specific allergens or animal products, or to seek out ingredients that could potentially deliver the effects you want. An ingredient list that doesn't follow regulations can indicate that the brand isn't familiar with industry standards and legal requirements, so is best avoided.

What doesn't it tell us?

Ingredient lists don't reveal everything about the product. This is intentional, as companies don't want their competitors to know exactly how they made their product. Plus they won't tell you how well products work. It's a lot like cooking – a well-cooked meal can have the exact same ingredients as a poorly prepared one. How the ingredients are combined is crucial to both how a dish interacts with your taste buds, and how a beauty product interacts with your body.

A single ingredient name can be used for many different materials. In particular, natural ingredients with the same name can have very different compositions and effects depending on factors like cultivation and processing methods. Synthetic materials can vary too – for example, "cetearyl alcohol" is a mixture of cetyl and stearyl alcohols, but their concentrations aren't fixed.

An ingredient might be in a special delivery system that makes it work more effectively. For example, an unstable ingredient might be wrapped in a protective coating. However, the ingredient and coating material will be listed as if they were introduced into the product separately.

CAN I FIND OUT THE EXACT QUANTITIES OF INGREDIENTS?

Companies don't always disclose the amounts of ingredients used. However, one clue for working out some ingredient concentrations is known as the "1% line".

Some ingredients are almost always used in quantities below 1%, including some preservatives (phenoxyethanol, benzoic acid), pH adjusters (sodium hydroxide, citric acid), and fragrance. Ingredients listed after these are most likely also present in quantities under 1% – but this isn't a guarantee.

Ingredient names
Standardized names from the International Nomenclature of Cosmetic Ingredients (INCI) are used.

Order of ingredients
Ingredients are listed in descending order by weight, starting with those present at higher concentrations. Ingredients included below 1% can be listed in any order.

Botanical ingredients
Listed using their Latin names.

Colouring agents
Can be listed separately, after "May contain" or "+/-" in any order.

Directions for use and storage
How the product should be used, and stored to prevent early expiry.

Batch number and expiry date
Which batch the product is from, for quality control and recall purposes, and how long the product is expected to work as advertised.

DIRECTIONS:
Apply liberally to dry skin daily. Store below 30°C.

LOT MW2388
EXP 02/2028

Brand Name, 101 Park Avenue, London EC1A

BRAND NAME

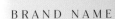

BODY
LOTION

100 ml e

12M

INGREDIENTS: Aqua, Caprylic/ Capric Triglyceride, Glycerin, Cetearyl Alcohol, Ceteareth-20, Prunus Amygdalus Dulcis (Sweet Almond) Oil, Tocopherol, Xanthan Gum, Phenoxyethanol, Ethylhexylglycerin, Citric Acid, Fragrance, Linalool.

Contact details
For further information, or to report adverse events.

Fragrances
Can be listed as "fragrance" or "parfum". In some regions, common fragrance allergens are listed separately if present at concentrations that could cause allergic reactions.

Flavours
Can be listed as "flavour" or "aroma".

Product size
Weight or volume of product inside the container. An "e" mark indicates that the size complies with relevant European laws.

Period after opening (PAO)
How long (in months) the product should stay safe to use after it is first opened, if stored under recommended conditions.

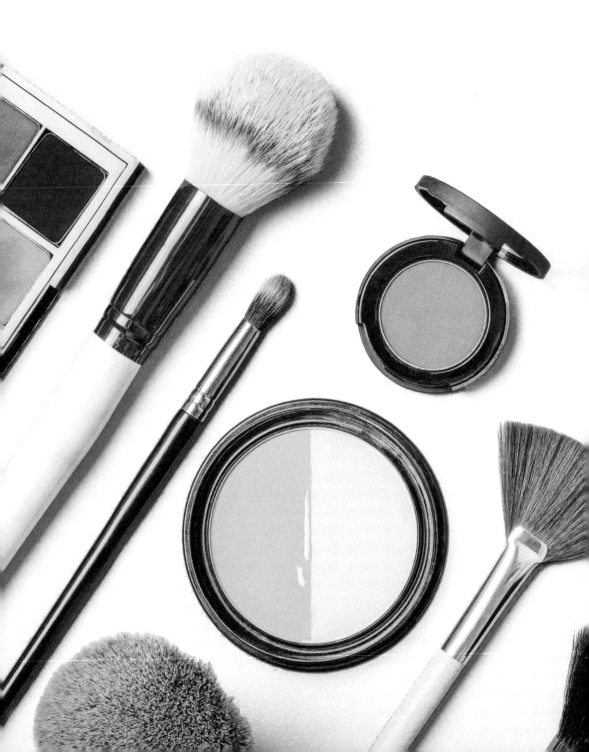

How should I store my beauty products?

You've probably had a beauty product go off at some point. It might have changed colour, smell, or texture, or grown a spot of mould. Some changes are harmless, but it often means the product is no longer safe or effective. Storage instructions are usually shown on the label, but here are a few tips to keep your products at their best for as long as possible.

Store products in a cool place as heat can cause ingredients to break down and emulsions to separate. Sunscreens are particularly sensitive to high temperatures. Many microbes also multiply faster in warm conditions. Most products will last longer if refrigerated, but freezing usually causes separation.

Store products away from light as it can also decompose many ingredients like sunscreens, fragrances, skincare actives, and natural extracts. Opaque packaging is often used to protect sensitive products.

Keep containers closed when not in use as oxygen can oxidize many ingredients, and any air or water going into the product can introduce microbes. Avoid using products in humid bathrooms.

Keep products in their original packaging as products can react with packaging materials, so compatibility is tested before manufacture. For example, many sunscreens can react with plastics, acids can corrode metal springs, and silicone hair products can react with silicone packaging.

Packaging is often carefully chosen to protect the specific formula. Coloured or opaque packaging blocks light, while packaging with less room for air can reduce exposure to oxygen. Transferring a product to different packaging can also expose it to a lot of oxygen and microbes in the air.

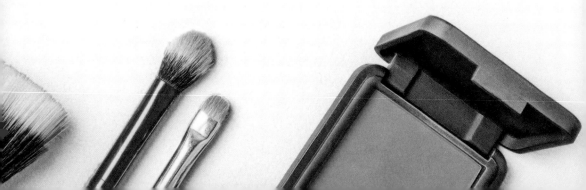

Can beauty products be sustainable?

The environmental impacts of everyday products are a hot topic. Consumers are increasingly willing to pay a premium for more sustainable products, but it can be difficult to figure out what is and isn't greenwashing.

When viewed holistically from a life cycle perspective, many product claims that seem eco-friendly have hidden downsides that can outweigh their benefits. Consumers tend to prioritize end-of-life considerations like recyclable packaging and biodegradability, even though these are not necessarily the biggest impacts. Sustainability needs to be evaluated on a case-by-case basis. Here are some common greenwashing assumptions in marketing:

"NATURAL INGREDIENTS ARE ALWAYS BETTER FOR THE ENVIRONMENT."

Natural ingredients are often assumed to be less impactful than synthetic ones. Here are some examples that highlight the inaccuracy of any blanket statements.

Wild ingredients
Unsustainable exploitation of natural resources is a problem, e.g. high demand for sandalwood oil has endangered wild trees, and overharvesting of wild licorice contributes to desertification.

Fossil fuel use
Synthetic ingredients from petrochemicals are not necessarily less eco-friendly, since they come from waste, and petroleum extraction is driven by fuel consumption. Producing natural ingredients also usually uses fossil fuels. However, "upcycled" natural ingredients made from byproducts or wastes from other processes often have lower impacts.

End-of-life
Natural ingredients are not necessarily safer for wildlife. For example, zinc oxide is more toxic for many aquatic organisms than most chemical sunscreens (although current evidence indicates that sunscreens do not have a significant impact on coral reefs).

Farmed ingredients
Farming can reduce strain on natural resources, but it has large impacts like deforestation, water pollution, and high energy use. Using land to farm cosmetic ingredients can also be unethical in the context of food insecurity.

Biotechnology
Plant cell cultures and genetic engineering can use nature's machinery to produce ingredients with far lower impacts, but many techniques are considered "unnatural".

"PLASTIC IS THE WORST OPTION FOR PACKAGING"

Plastic is often not the most environmentally damaging option for packaging when steps aside from end-of-life are considered. Again, the best option depends on the specific circumstances.

Transport
Plastic is strong for its weight so its transport produces less carbon emissions than glass. Glass also often breaks during transport so there is greater loss of product. Aluminium containers tend to dent easily, making them difficult to sell.

Production
Newly manufactured plastic is mostly made from waste materials from fuel production. First-use paper production requires wood, while aluminium and glass require a lot more heat. Depending on the application, these can all be produced from recycled sources as well.

End-of-life
Plastic has more downsides when it comes to end-of-life – glass and aluminium can be recycled more times, while paper is very biodegradable. However, since paper doesn't stand up to water, it's often lined with plastic. This makes it far more difficult to recycle than monomaterial plastic. Beauty packaging components can also be small and difficult to recycle.

"Eco-friendly" packaging
Glass, aluminium, and paper packaging are often assumed to be automatically better than plastic, but they have less obvious drawbacks.

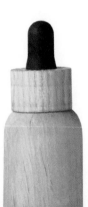
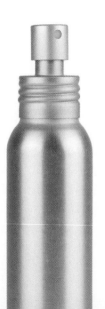
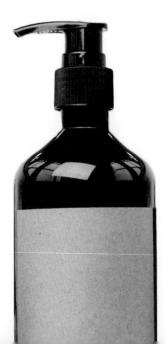

Raw materials
Impacts associated with obtaining the raw materials, like mining or farming. Multiple raw materials can be used for a single ingredient.

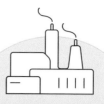

Processing
Materials are processed to create the product components. This includes purification and synthesis. The same ingredient can be processed in many ways, with different impacts.

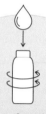

Manufacturing
Processed materials are transformed into the final product. Identical formulas can have different impacts, such as if one manufacturer uses renewable energy.

Disposal and recycling (end-of-life)
Where the product and packaging go after use. We often focus on this stage, since it's what we can see and control, even though it might not contribute much to the overall impact.

LIFE CYCLE ASSESSMENT

Consumer use
This can be significant for some products e.g. energy to heat shower water can be the largest contributor to a shampoo's environmental impact.

Distribution and transport
Finished products are transported to distributors, retailers, and consumers.

Life cycle assessment

Many initiatives that seem environmentally friendly will just shift the impact to a different stage. A life cycle assessment (LCA) can prevent this from happening by quantifying all the environmental impacts at each step of a beauty product's life. This includes the production and processing of each raw material (in both product and packaging), manufacturing, distribution, consumer use, and disposal and recycling.

LCAs are complex since cosmetic products are usually made of many components. However, they are essential tools for establishing a baseline for impact reduction, guiding product development choices, and supporting environmental claims. There are ongoing efforts towards standardizing LCA methodologies so that products can be compared fairly.

BEAUTY MYTHS

"CARBON OFFSETS CANCEL OUT CARBON EMISSIONS"

Carbon offsets – where the planet-warming carbon dioxide emitted when making a product is "cancelled out" by investing in a carbon capture project – are problematic. Carbon capture projects would often have proceeded regardless of the donation, many projects do not eventuate, and there are many examples where offsets have been double-counted. The idea that they "cancel" can also create complacency, which hinders progress towards reducing emissions in the original process.

How to be more sustainable

It's tempting to think we can save the planet by making easy swaps in our beauty routines, but it really isn't that simple. Here are some tips for actually making your beauty routine more sustainable:

Consume less
It's rare that buying a beauty product is more environmentally friendly than not buying it. Think about whether you really need a product before purchasing.

Ask brands for evidence
Since sustainability is so context-dependent, it's impossible to work out if a brand has good evidence to back up their claims unless they provide some level of transparency.

Recycle thoughtfully
Not all materials and container sizes are accepted in standard kerbside recycling – you need to check for your location. Resin identification codes show the type of plastic used in a container; these are not recycling symbols. Some common plastics used for cosmetics include:

Polyethylene terephthalate
Used for most rigid transparent bottles, which are typically recyclable.

PET

High-density polyethylene
A tough plastic used for rigid containers and sacks.

HDPE

Polypropylene
Resists repeated bending. Used for most flip-top caps, pumps, and spray heads.

PP

Are my beauty products cruelty-free?

"Cruelty-free" usually means a product hasn't been tested on live animals. Animal testing of cosmetic products and ingredients has been rare for many years, but it's a complex situation, and products you personally consider "cruelty-free" may not be for someone else.

Why are tests done on animals?

The biology of a living organism is complicated, so it can be hard to predict how an ingredient or product might affect a human being or an animal. Humans share biological similarities with many animals, so animal tests have been used for centuries to approximate human impacts, with varying degrees of success. Stringent animal testing became mandatory for many industries from the 1930s, after several inadequately tested foods and drugs caused many injuries and deaths.

Since then, we have made considerable progress in understanding how substances act to cause harm. Some animal tests have been replaced with alternatives that mimic key steps in biological pathways (see Testing potential skin allergens, next page).

Many tests were developed by the cosmetics industry as a response to

ALTERNATIVES TO ANIMAL TESTING

Many tests can be used to predict whether a substance will harm humans, minimizing the need for animal testing in the future.

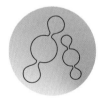

Inherent properties
A chemical's structure can determine how it interacts with the body.

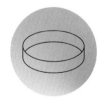

In vitro tests
How the substance affects cells or biological molecules like enzymes.

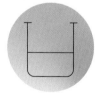

Artificial tissues
Cells can be cultured on 3D scaffolds to more closely mimic living tissue, then used in tests.

ethical concerns, pressure from animal welfare activists, and animal testing bans. These tests are often also cheaper, faster, and can give more accurate predictions of what happens in humans. Their use has been expanding to other areas outside of cosmetics.

However, many gaps remain. Reliable animal-free tests have not yet been developed for some complex biological processes. It is also harder to assess classes of ingredients that behave less predictably, or do not have historical animal testing data. Many regulators have also been slow to accept substitutes for animal tests.

Bans on animal testing for cosmetics

Cosmetics have only ever represented a very small fraction of animals used in scientific tests (only 0.04% in the EU in 1996, before any animal testing bans). However, it has been the focus of much publicity,

and regulations around the world have been rapidly evolving. Testing of cosmetic products and ingredients on animals was banned in the UK in 1998. In the European Union, animal testing of cosmetic products was banned in 2004, followed by cosmetic ingredients in 2009, while the marketing of any cosmetic products or ingredients tested on animals was banned in 2013.

China has long required animal testing for particular categories of cosmetics from foreign countries, but dropped mandatory animal testing for most domestically produced cosmetics in 2014, for select imported cosmetics in 2018, then for most imported cosmetics in 2021. These changes were in part due to the efforts of cosmetic companies operating in China, who worked with authorities to validate alternative tests.

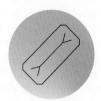

Organ chips
Different cell types are linked with microscopic channels to simulate living organs.

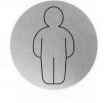

Clinical studies
Small amounts of substances are given to volunteers to trace how they behave in the body.

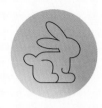

Existing data
Information from past animal studies can be used to evaluate similar substances.

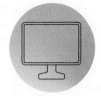

Computer models
Data from different sources are combined in computer models to predict biological activity.

What does cruelty-free mean?

There is no universal definition for "cruelty-free", beyond the fact that a specific *product* was not tested on animals. While most standards agree that *ingredients* should no longer be tested on animals solely for use in cosmetics, almost every ingredient would've been tested on animals at some point – by research scientists, to assess environmental or occupational safety, if the ingredient is used in other products, or before animal testing bans. Most regulators also have the right to test products on the market for safety, which can include animal tests. It's also worth bearing in mind that:

• Some in vitro tests still use animal-derived components such as animal skin or tissues, which can be from food industry waste, or animals bred and euthanized specifically for experiments.
• Some tests on early life stage organisms, such as fish embryos, are not counted as animal tests.
• "Cruelty-free" does not cover human rights concerns, like child labour or worker safety.
• "Cruelty-free" also does not necessarily mean vegan (free from ingredients sourced from animals).
• Products may still have been tested on animals by organizations other than the manufacturer, such as research scientists and government agencies.

TESTING POTENTIAL SKIN ALLERGENS

Instead of animal testing, alternative tests can be combined to predict ingredient safety. For example, the steps on the left need to occur for an ingredient to cause skin allergies. In step 2, the ingredient binds to specific proteins on skin. If it doesn't bind to these proteins in a test tube, it's unlikely to be an allergen.

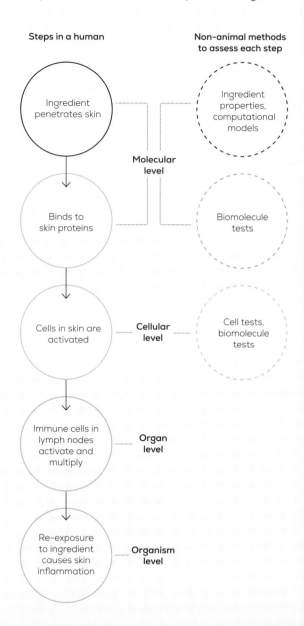

Steps in a human

Non-animal methods to assess each step

Ingredient penetrates skin

Ingredient properties, computational models

Molecular level

Binds to skin proteins

Biomolecule tests

Cells in skin are activated — Cellular level

Cell tests, biomolecule tests

Immune cells in lymph nodes activate and multiply — Organ level

Re-exposure to ingredient causes skin inflammation — Organism level

How does menopause affect my hair and skin?

While many aspects of skin and hair change as we get older, some are specifically related to the hormonal shifts brought about by menopause.

At menopause, the ovaries stop producing oestrogen and progesterone, which causes changes in skin and hair.

Skin

Lower oestrogen leads to loss of collagen in the lower layer of skin (dermis), which can decrease by 30% in the first 5 years after menopause. As a result, skin becomes thinner and less firm, with more noticeable fine lines and blood vessels. Skin cell production slows, leading to a thinner skin barrier. Lower progesterone also reduces oil production. Skin becomes less hydrated with a dry, rough texture, and can feel itchy and tight. Reduced oestrogen is also linked to impaired wound healing after menopause.

Studies have observed that hormone replacement therapy can prevent or even reverse some of these skin changes. However, the skin benefits alone are generally not enough to warrant starting treatment.

Hair

Some studies have found that hair fibre diameter, density, and growth decrease after menopause, particularly near the forehead. Lowered oil production means hair is usually less greasy after menopause, but also less shiny and soft.

Some hair changes linked to aging aren't directly linked to menopause, but tend to occur around the same time. These include female pattern hair loss and increased facial hair.

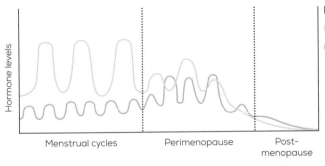

Hormone levels

Menstrual cycles   Perimenopause   Post-menopause

Key

Progesterone

Oestrogen

Hormone fluctuations

Oestrogen and progesterone levels change over time, from the regular peaks and troughs of the menstrual cycle, to the unpredictable fluctuations and decline from perimenopause onwards.

How does pregnancy affect my hair and skin?

Many hormonal, immune, and anatomical changes occur during pregnancy, which can be reflected in skin, hair, and nails. These usually reverse after childbirth.

Be aware that some changes can indicate health problems, and should be mentioned to your doctor. Here are some of the most common changes you're likely to experience when pregnant.

Skin changes

Pigmented areas like moles, nipples, and genitals often darken during pregnancy. **Irregular patches of melasma** often develop on the cheeks, nose, and forehead during the latter half of pregnancy, especially in darker skin. This is caused by higher oestrogen and progesterone levels, and darkens with sun exposure.

Sebum (skin oil) production increases due to rising androgen levels, which can exacerbate acne.
Small red veins might appear on the upper body, while swollen varicose veins can occur in the legs and pelvic area due to reduced blood flow. Moving around regularly and putting your feet up can help.
Stretch marks (striae gravidarum) often form on the stomach, breasts, and upper thighs as the baby grows. They usually start off reddish or purple, then turn white (see p124). Skin can also become sensitive and rashes can develop.

Hair and nail changes

Both head and body hair often grow faster and thicker. After birth, there can be increased hair loss as excess hair sheds and growth returns to normal.

Nails often grow faster during pregnancy and can become brittle, split, and break.

What products do I need to avoid during pregnancy?

A few ingredients and products can harm developing babies, who may be exposed through the placenta. However, like many other "pregnancy rules", a lot of concerns are overstated. Most cosmetic products absorb minimally into the body, so are considered safe during pregnancy. Safety assessments consider use by pregnant people.

- Unbranded, illegally imported, or potentially counterfeit products from

Most cosmetic products absorb minimally into the body, so are considered safe during pregnancy.

dubious sources are not recommended as they may not meet safety standards.

- Hydroquinone is not recommended.
- Retinoids (vitamin A derivatives) in skincare are usually not recommended during pregnancy as a precaution due to the risks of oral isotretinoin, which can cause birth defects. However, retinoids do not absorb easily into blood and skincare only contains small amounts, so the risk is expected to be very low. If you have accidentally used a retinoid, there is no need to panic.

Check with your doctors and local health authorities for up-to-date advice, and consult your doctor before stopping any medications.

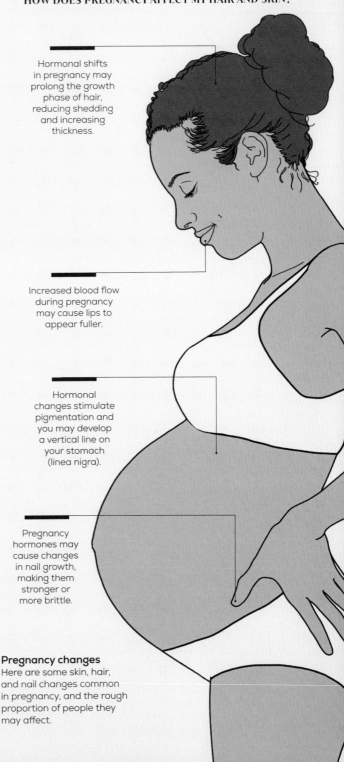

Hormonal shifts in pregnancy may prolong the growth phase of hair, reducing shedding and increasing thickness.

Increased blood flow during pregnancy may cause lips to appear fuller.

Hormonal changes stimulate pigmentation and you may develop a vertical line on your stomach (linea nigra).

Pregnancy hormones may cause changes in nail growth, making them stronger or more brittle.

Pregnancy changes
Here are some skin, hair, and nail changes common in pregnancy, and the rough proportion of people they may affect.

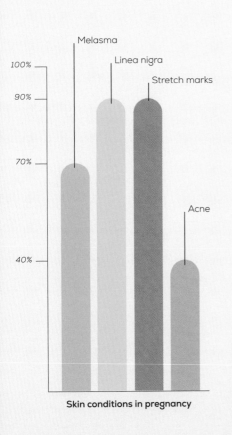

Melasma

Linea nigra

Stretch marks

Acne

100%

90%

70%

40%

Skin conditions in pregnancy

Everyday skincare

What is skin?

Our skin is a complex but elegant barrier between us and the outside world. It mainly acts as protection, but also allows us to communicate with and respond to our environment.

The skin is made up of three main layers: epidermis, dermis, and hypodermis (see diagram opposite).

Epidermis

The epidermis sits at the top and functions mainly as a physical barrier. It prevents microorganisms and environmental substances from entering, and essential skin components (like water) from escaping.

The topmost layer of epidermis – the skin we see and touch – is the stratum corneum. This is a waterproof layer of dead skin cells surrounded by oily substances called lipids. Each cell is made up of keratin and water-binding substances (called the natural moisturizing factor), encased in a tough shell of proteins and lipids. It is usually around 15 cell layers deep, but can be thicker in areas that need more protection, like palms and knees. We shed around one layer of these cells each day, with the entire stratum corneum being replaced every two weeks or so – a process called desquamation.

The bottom (basal) layer of the epidermis contains adult stem cells. These divide to produce the keratinocyte cells that eventually form the stratum corneum, pushing upwards and replenishing the layers that are shed. Along the way they flatten out, die, lose water, and release lipids for the stratum corneum. Keratinocytes also produce antioxidants that protect against free radicals formed by oxygen, pollutants, and UV. The epidermis is also where melanin pigment and vitamin D are produced.

Dermis

The dermis lies under the epidermis, and gives skin much of its elasticity, strength, and flexibility. It contains a network of protein fibres, mostly collagen and elastin. These are surrounded by a gel containing hyaluronic acid, which binds enormous quantities of water.

Blood vessels in the dermis transport nutrients, dilate or contract to regulate heat loss, and contribute to skin colour. Nerve endings sense pain, touch, and temperature. Hair follicles originate in the dermis, and open to the skin's surface to form pores. Sebaceous glands inside hair follicles produce sebum (skin oil).

Sweat glands in the dermis produce sweat in response to heat or stress. Sebum and sweat create a slightly acidic waterproof coating on the skin's surface called the acid mantle. It helps maintain the balance of microorganisms (skin microbiome) and provides lubrication.

Hypodermis

Below the dermis is the hypodermis or subcutaneous layer, which contains fat and connective tissue. It acts as shock absorber, energy store, and thermal insulation.

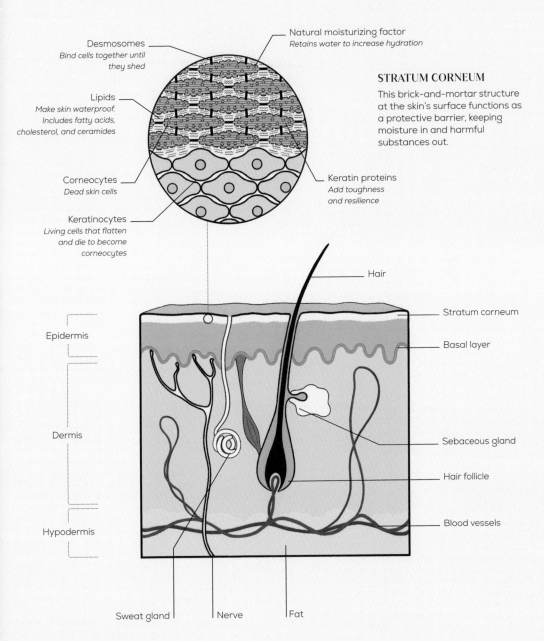

Desmosomes
Bind cells together until they shed

Natural moisturizing factor
Retains water to increase hydration

STRATUM CORNEUM

This brick-and-mortar structure at the skin's surface functions as a protective barrier, keeping moisture in and harmful substances out.

Lipids
Make skin waterproof. Includes fatty acids, cholesterol, and ceramides

Corneocytes
Dead skin cells

Keratin proteins
Add toughness and resilience

Keratinocytes
Living cells that flatten and die to become corneocytes

Hair

Stratum corneum

Basal layer

Epidermis

Dermis

Sebaceous gland

Hair follicle

Blood vessels

Hypodermis

Sweat gland

Nerve

Fat

STRUCTURE OF SKIN

Each layer of the skin plays an important role, from the protective epidermis to the supportive dermis, and the fat-storing hypodermis.

Why do we even need skincare?

Skin has largely evolved to take care of itself, but our environment has drastically changed. Temperature, humidity, sun exposure, hormones, and even skincare and grooming habits can disrupt its function.

On top of this, evolution favours features that help humans survive long enough to reproduce and pass on their genes. It doesn't necessarily help our skin feel comfortable, or function optimally.

Skincare products, including both medical and cosmetic products, can make up for what skin can't do on its own. They can protect against environmental insults, replenish skin's components, and treat skin disorders. Skin experts from all fields largely agree that most people should be using cleanser, moisturizer, and sunscreen, regardless of gender or skin type.

As well as maintaining optimal physiological function, skincare products can also change the skin's appearance. Skin is translucent, so smoothing, hydrating, and compacting the outer layers leads to more reflected light, making skin appear more radiant.

Skincare products can prevent and even reverse structural changes that occur with aging, although the effects are largely limited to the more superficial layers. Some products can help smooth lines and wrinkles, and even out skin tone and pigmentation.

Cleansers and moisturizers are key products in any skincare routine.

Cleanser

Cleansers remove unwanted substances from skin. This includes pollutants, makeup, and microbes that might cause infection

Most people should be using cleanser, moisturizer, and sunscreen, regardless of gender or skin type.

or disease. It also removes dead cells, sweat, and sebum, which can contribute to clogged pores.

Moisturizer

Moisturizers make up for lack of water or oil in the stratum corneum, and can improve its ability to act as a barrier. Many biological processes in skin react to how well the skin barrier is functioning, so moisturizers can have longer-term effects. For example, lack of water causes irregular shedding of cells, leading to rough and flaky skin. "Inert" petroleum jelly has been found to increase the skin's production of antimicrobial peptides. In elderly people, moisturizers have been found to decrease inflammatory markers in blood, which could potentially improve inflammation-dependent conditions like cognitive decline.

How to choose skincare products

Because skincare products and skin are so variable, there isn't really a substitute for trying out products on your skin. You can narrow down product choices by looking at reviews from people with a similar skin type and concerns to you, and check claims and ingredients (pp34–37).

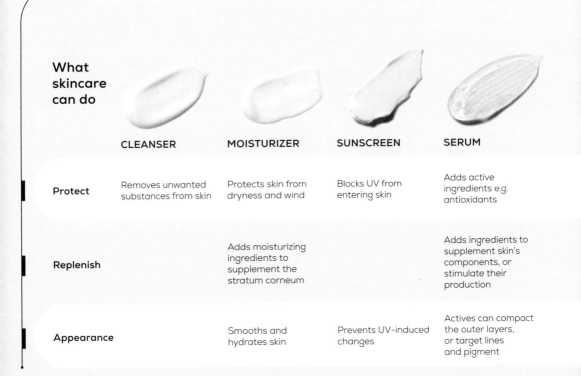

What skincare can do

	CLEANSER	MOISTURIZER	SUNSCREEN	SERUM
Protect	Removes unwanted substances from skin	Protects skin from dryness and wind	Blocks UV from entering skin	Adds active ingredients e.g. antioxidants
Replenish		Adds moisturizing ingredients to supplement the stratum corneum		Adds ingredients to supplement skin's components, or stimulate their production
Appearance		Smooths and hydrates skin	Prevents UV-induced changes	Actives can compact the outer layers, or target lines and pigment

How do I choose a cleanser?

Cleansers remove unwanted substances including dirt, sebum, microorganisms, and skincare products that could otherwise clog pores and impact skin function.

Many of these substances are oily, so they cannot be dissolved by water alone. Cleansers contain surfactants (see below), which bind to oils and allow them to be rinsed away.

Cleansing surfactants

Surfactants are classified by the charge of the head. Three categories are in cleansers:
- Anionic surfactants (e.g. soaps, sulfates, and taurates) have negatively charged heads.
- Amphoteric surfactants (including betaines and amphoacetates) can have both positive and negative charges.
- Non-ionic surfactants (such as PEG oils and glucosides) have uncharged heads.

Most cleansers contain a mix of all three types. Anionic surfactants are used for their cleaning and foaming abilities, while amphoteric and non-ionic surfactants are added to decrease irritation, and adjust the texture of the product and foam.

The importance of gentle cleansing

While surfactants are necessary, they can remove skin's natural proteins and lipids, and stay attached to skin after rinsing. This disturbs the barrier, causing dryness and

HOW SURFACTANTS CLEAN

Clever little cleaning agents, surfactants work by attaching their hydrophobic tails to contaminants while their hydrophilic heads enable them to disperse in water, so dirt can be rinsed away.

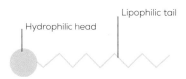

Hydrophilic head

Lipophilic tail

Surfactant molecule
The tail binds to oil, while the head prefers water.

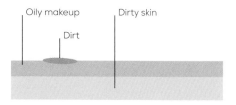

Oily makeup

Dirt

Dirty skin

1 Ready to cleanse
It's the end of another day of wearing oily makeup and battling the elements. Dirt and oil on your skin need to be removed.

irritation. To combat this, cleansers are increasingly formulated to be gentler. All skin types benefit from gentle cleansing, so look for products containing:

- Multiple surfactants, which form clusters that keep individual surfactants out of the skin.
- Polymers, which can hold onto surfactants so they're not left behind.
- Moisturizing ingredients like oils and glycerin.
- Soothing ingredients like antioxidants, niacinamide, and allantoin.

Cleansers with a slightly acidic pH of 4–6 are particularly helpful for acne-prone and sensitive skin, as they support a healthy skin microbiome.

Should I avoid sulfates?

Sodium lauryl sulfate (SLS) and sodium laureth sulfate (SLES) are surfactants with a reputation for being harsh and stripping. This isn't necessarily true. While SLS's narrow structure penetrates skin more easily, SLES is milder than many other surfactants. Mildness formulating techniques are also used to make sulfate-containing cleansers gentler. Reviews of specific cleansers will give a more accurate idea of how gentle they are than just the presence or absence of sulfates.

Should I avoid foaming cleansers?

Older cleansers used high concentrations of SLS to create foam, which could be harsh. But modern foaming cleansers aren't necessarily harsh, thanks to newer surfactants and mildness-boosting formulation techniques. In one study, a non-foaming cleanser was more drying than a foaming cleanser with added moisturizers. Additionally, ingredients like glycerin and thickeners can stabilize foam without increasing irritation.

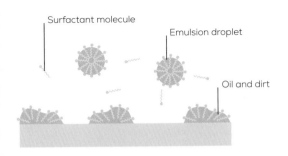

Surfactant molecule
Emulsion droplet
Oil and dirt

2 Add water and cleanser
Surfactants to the rescue! They lift oil and dirt from skin, suspending them in water for easy removal.

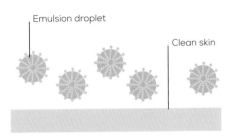

Emulsion droplet
Clean skin

3 Clean skin
The dirt and oils have been rinsed away, leaving skin cleansed. You're looking fresh and radiant once again!

Do I need to moisturize?

Moisturizers add water or oil to the stratum corneum, to relieve flaking, dullness, and loss of flexibility.

Moisturizing is essential for maintaining healthy skin. As well as promoting a smooth, radiant complexion, it supports the skin's natural barrier function, protecting it from environmental stressors.

Occlusives
These form a water-repellent layer that reduces the natural evaporation of water from skin (transepidermal water loss or TEWL). Examples include petroleum jelly, mineral oil, and dimethicone.

Emollients
These oily ingredients make skin smoother, softer, and more lubricated. They include plant oils and butters, fatty esters (e.g. C12-15 alkyl benzoate), fatty alcohols (e.g. cetyl alcohol), silicones, ceramides, and squalane. Many occlusives are also emollients.

Humectants

These bind to water to slow its evaporation. Examples include glycerin, urea, glycols, and hyaluronic acid. They can feel sticky if too much is used.

HOW DO I CHOOSE A MOISTURIZER?

In studies, some moisturizers actually dried skin out, potentially because other ingredients like emulsifiers were disturbing the skin barrier. Look for clinical evidence, choose a brand that tests their formulas, and check reviews.

Using other products too?
Many skincare products contain moisturizing ingredients, so you might not need a separate moisturizer.

Do you have dry skin?
Dry skin benefits from all three moisturizer categories (see left).

Do you have oily skin?
Oily skin prone to dehydration benefits most from humectants and occlusives (occlusives may be too shiny for daytime use).

Is your skin balanced?
Skin with enough oil and water might not need moisturizer – using one can even signal to the skin to produce less of its own moisturizing components.

Check the ingredient list
The moisturizer types in the first five ingredients will give an indication of whether it'll suit your skin.

Consider the texture
Moisturizer texture is adjusted using thickeners and might not reflect its richness. But by convention, moisturizers designed for dry skin are usually thicker, while those for oily skin are more lightweight.

Moisturizing ingredients
These three major ingredient categories act in different ways to moisturize skin.

What is my skin type?

Skin type is a broad way of categorizing the amount of oil your skin produces. It can help you identify the products that best address your skincare goals.

Skin type is mostly determined by genetics and hormones, but temporary changes like stress, diet, weather, humidity, and the products you use can exacerbate dryness or oiliness. Oil production tends to slow with age (see pp64–65), and can be reduced by medications such as spironolactone and hormonal contraceptives.

Skincare routine for dry skin

1. Cleanser Use a gentle cleanser that includes oils, like a cream cleanser, once or twice daily.
2. Moisturizer Look for well-rounded moisturizers with occlusives, emollients, and humectants to add oil and water back to skin.
3. Sunscreen Most sunscreens are moisturizing, but you may need to layer a moisturizer underneath.

Skincare routine for oily skin

1. Cleanser Use a gentle gel or foaming cleanser once or twice daily. Some cleansers can help soak up oil with ingredients like clay.
2. Moisturizer A gel moisturizer or toner containing humectants can hydrate skin in dry weather. You may not need to moisturize every day, or you may only need to moisturize certain parts of your skin.
3. Sunscreen Look for fluid or gel formulas designed to be lightweight on oily skin.

For combination skin, customize your routine so you're treating oily areas with products formulated for oil control, while moisturizing dry areas as needed. Any routine involving a gentle cleanser and sunscreen is usually sufficient to maintain "normal" skin.

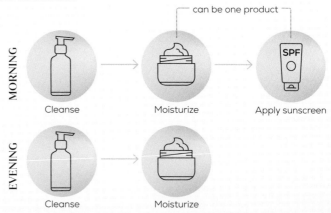

can be one product

MORNING
Cleanse → Moisturize → Apply sunscreen

EVENING
Cleanse → Moisturize

A basic skincare routine
Your skincare regimen can become as complicated as you'd like. But to begin with, you need these basic steps.

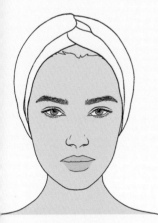

Normal skin
"Normal" or balanced
skin produces a moderate
amount of oil.

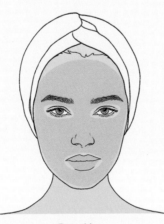

Dry skin
Doesn't look shiny, not many
visible pores. Often feels tight.
Tends to feel better with
moisturizer. Prone to flakes
and rough patches. Makeup
settles into fine lines.

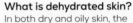

- **What is dehydrated skin?**
In both dry and oily skin, the
stratum corneum's water
content can drop below the
20–30% needed for optimal
function. Skin cells shrink,
leading to flaking and cracking.
This can cause oily skin to feel
paradoxically dry and oily at
the same time. Skin might feel
tight after washing, and
temporary wrinkles and fine
lines from water loss form.

- **What is sensitive skin?**
Sensitive skin reacts easily
to environmental triggers like
jewellery, fragrance, laundry
detergents, water exposure,
and heat. It often stings,
itches, swells, feels hot, or
develops rashes. There is
often a weakened skin barrier,
which lets in more irritants,
along with a hyperactive
inflammatory response.
Sensitivity can be related to
conditions like rosacea, atopic
dermatitis, and allergies.

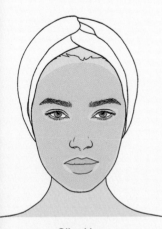

Oily skin
Shiny patches of oil. Doesn't
need much moisturizer, except
in very dry weather. Prone to
enlarged and clogged pores,
especially in the T-zone.
Makeup slides around.

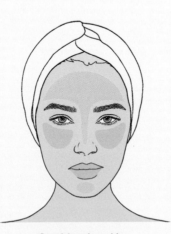

Combination skin
Skin has areas which fall under
different categories. The cheeks are
usually drier, while the "T-zone"
(forehead, nose, and chin)
produces more oil.

DIFFERENT SKIN TYPES
Understanding your skin
type is crucial for choosing
products and routines tailored
to your skin's specific needs.

What happens to skin as we age?

Our skin undergoes noticeable changes at different stages of life, which affects how we can best take care of it.

Infants

Baby skin is thinner with a weaker barrier, so it is more prone to dryness, irritation, and sunburn. 1 in 5 babies have atopic dermatitis, compared to 1 in 30 adults. By age 5, barrier function is similar to adults. However, studies indicate that cells may be more vulnerable to UV during childhood, so excessive sun exposure in youth can magnify melanoma risk.

Adolescents

During puberty, increased testosterone causes a surge in sebum. This changes the skin microbiome and clogs pores, which can trigger conditions like acne and dandruff. Apocrine sweat glands start to secrete lipids and peptides, which are metabolized by bacteria to create body odour. Skin changes related to the menstrual cycle begin. Rapid growth can lead to stretch marks.

Adults

As we grow older, internal and external changes affect our skin's function and appearance. Differences in appearance are completely normal, even though we've often been conditioned to see them as something to be fixed. However, changes in function will inform how best to take care of skin at different life stages.

Internal factors that impact skin over time are largely controlled by genetics. From about age 25, the skin's renewal and maintenance processes start to slow due to changes in hormone, immune, and repair systems. Skin components also accumulate free radical damage from regular bodily processes, while exposed areas like the face and hands are impacted by sunlight, smoking, and pollution. The skin barrier is drier, rougher, and more permeable with age, as cell renewal slows and becomes less uniform. All layers of the skin thin, becoming less elastic and more fragile.

Skin colour and race affect the visible changes that occur. Pigment changes like age spots dominate in East Asian skin until around age 40, followed by accelerated wrinkling, while texture changes like wrinkles tend to occur earlier in white skin. In addition to uneven pigment, darker skin can become ashy due to a thicker and rougher stratum corneum. Women usually have slower changes in texture than men until menopause, when rapidly declining oestrogen thins the skin and fat layers that soften the appearance of wrinkles.

How skin damage develops

Over time, many microscopic mechanisms contribute to damage that eventually shows up on the skin's surface. Decreased fat, muscle, and bone under the skin also contribute to visible changes.

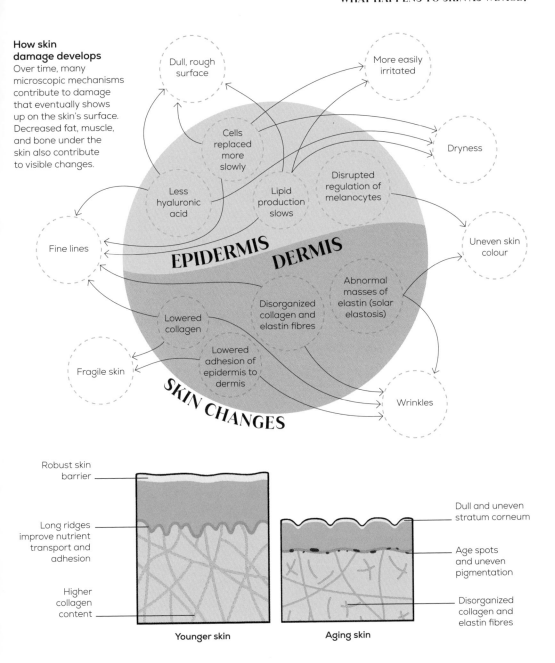

How skin ages

Some age-related changes in the skin's structure are shown here.

Younger skin

Aging skin

- Robust skin barrier
- Long ridges improve nutrient transport and adhesion
- Higher collagen content

- Dull and uneven stratum corneum
- Age spots and uneven pigmentation
- Disorganized collagen and elastin fibres

Should I change my skincare routine?

It's easy to keep using the same products day after day – after all, it's called a routine for a reason.

However, as seasons change and our hormones fluctuate, there are benefits to making a change.

Climate and weather

Skin loses water more quickly when it's dry and windy, which can warrant more moisturizing. Artificial heating and long hot showers will further dry out skin. Sun protection becomes more important in spring and summer. Moving countries or travelling can also impact skin – as well as a different climate, you may experience changes in diet, water quality, air pollution, stress, and sleep.

Age

The skin's needs evolve as we age. Baby skin is sensitive, so gentle cleansers and moisturizers are recommended. Common food allergens should be avoided in skincare as they can increase the risk of developing food allergies. Sun protection is especially important in childhood – for babies, sun protective clothing and shade are recommended over sunscreen.

During puberty, sebaceous glands become more active, causing oilier skin. This is when many people start using skincare products, particularly cleansers and clay masks to remove oil. Over-the-counter treatments containing salicylic acid and benzoyl peroxide can be helpful for acne, while more severe cases may need prescription treatments.

Skin becomes drier and more fragile with advancing age, so gentle cleansers and moisturizers are important.

Does skin get used to skincare products?

Aside from antibiotics, there's little evidence that other skincare products become less effective over time and need to be changed periodically. The effects of skincare products do tend to be most noticeable when you start using them and can become less obvious over time, but skin will usually revert to its original condition after you stop.

SKINCARE DURING YOUR MENSTRUAL CYCLE

While the menstrual cycle doesn't affect everyone's skin, some people might need different skincare products throughout the month. These are the most common changes.

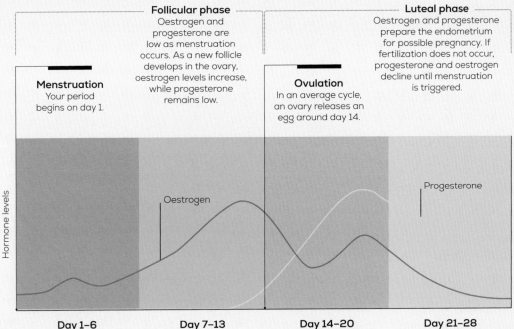

Follicular phase
Oestrogen and progesterone are low as menstruation occurs. As a new follicle develops in the ovary, oestrogen levels increase, while progesterone remains low.

Luteal phase
Oestrogen and progesterone prepare the endometrium for possible pregnancy. If fertilization does not occur, progesterone and oestrogen decline until menstruation is triggered.

Menstruation
Your period begins on day 1.

Ovulation
In an average cycle, an ovary releases an egg around day 14.

Hormone levels

Oestrogen

Progesterone

Day 1–6
Skin is driest, so you may need to use more moisturizer.

Day 7–13
Skin is less oily, more hydrated and thicker, and usually looks its best. Start using acne products if you're prone to premenstrual flares.

Day 14–20
Sebum increases, so you may need less moisturizer. Oily skin may need shine control products.

Day 21–28
Skin may be more sensitive, so reduce any irritating products. Many conditions can flare, including acne.

Is face wash better than bar soap?

Some people swear by washing their face with a bar of soap, while others prefer liquid cleansers. While both contain surfactants, their specific ingredients differ.

"Soap" refers to cleansing surfactants made by reacting naturally occurring fats and oils with alkalis, like lye or caustic potash. Glycerin is a natural byproduct of the soap-making process, but is often removed to prevent soap bars from going mushy.

The shortage of edible fats and oils during World War I led to the development of synthetic surfactants, called "detergents". These became the predominant cleansing ingredients by the 1950s.

Soaps do not work well in hard water containing calcium and magnesium ions, which bind to soap's head groups to form gritty scum. They also stop working and turn oily in acidic water. However, detergents have different head groups, so they can tolerate these conditions and have a wider range of uses.

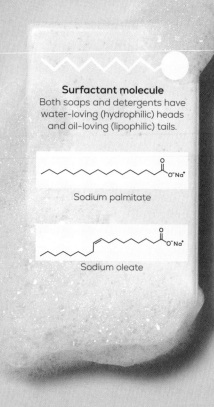

Surfactant molecule
Both soaps and detergents have water-loving (hydrophilic) heads and oil-loving (lipophilic) tails.

Sodium palmitate

Sodium oleate

Which one should I use?

Both solid and liquid cleansers can clean well, but the diverse properties of synthetic detergents mean liquid cleansers are usually more beneficial. Most bars contain natural soaps, which only work at high pH and disrupt the skin's acid mantle. Their narrow

SOLID SOAP

Solid fats and oils like tallow (beef fat), lard, and palm oil tend to produce harder soap bars, due to their high saturated fat content.

> The diverse properties of synthetic detergents mean liquid cleansers are usually more beneficial.

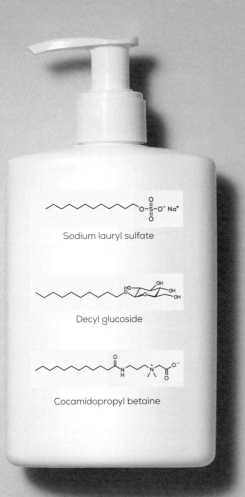

Sodium lauryl sulfate

Decyl glucoside

Cocamidopropyl betaine

LIQUID CLEANSER

Liquid cleansers usually contain synthetic detergents. Natural liquid soaps are made from liquid plant oils, which have more unsaturated fatty acids.

structures can burrow into skin and cause irritation. However, some bars use detergents like isethionates and have a more skin-friendly acidic pH.

Liquid cleansers usually contain synthetic detergents, which can work at a lower pH and have bulkier structures, leading to less barrier disturbance. There is also more flexibility for including beneficial skincare ingredients. However, some detergent-based formulas can still be harsh, and liquid cleansers that contain soap surfactants can have similar drawbacks to solid soaps.

What about other kinds of cleanser?

While you could technically clean your face with any kind of cleanser – body wash, shampoo, even washing-up liquid – they are formulated for different purposes, and are more likely to cause irritation. They will also contain ingredients specific to their function, such as amodimethicone, a detangling ingredient in shampoos that binds to the hair.

Do I need to exfoliate?

Most people can benefit from using an exfoliant. They can help with clogged pores, acne, dull and rough skin, uneven texture, or uneven skin tone.

Your skin naturally exfoliates itself, but many factors can disrupt this process, like humidity or aging. You can use an exfoliant once or twice a week to supplement the natural process. Exfoliants should be introduced gradually, as overuse can thin the stratum corneum too much and impair its barrier function, leading to sensitivity, tightness, and stinging.

Overuse of exfoliants can thin the stratum corneum too much and impair its barrier function, leading to sensitivity, tightness, and stinging.

Types of exfoliants

Exfoliants can be divided into two categories: physical and chemical (or enzyme).

Physical exfoliants work by mechanically buffing away surface cells. Intensity depends on pressure and application time. They include scrubs, peeling gels (gommages), and tools like brushes, cloths, and sponges. Scrub particles can be made of many materials such as cellulose, ground nut shells, wax beads, or sugar grains.

Chemical and enzyme exfoliants break dead cell layers into smaller pieces that detach more easily. Chemical exfoliants include alpha hydroxy acids (such as glycolic and lactic acids), salicylic acid (commonly called beta hydroxy acid), and polyhydroxy acids (including gluconolactone and lactobionic acid). Exfoliating enzymes are commonly sourced from fruits, and include bromelain (from pineapple), papain (from papaya), and actinidin (from kiwi fruit).

Choosing an exfoliant

Many people overuse physical exfoliants, so chemical or enzyme exfoliants are usually recommended instead, especially if you have sensitive skin. Using 5% alpha hydroxy acid or 2% salicylic acid twice a week is a good starting point.

What difference does a good night's sleep make?

Sleep is essential for good health – a fact that's as true for our skin as for any other part of our body.

Poor sleep shows on your face, and studies have found that you can appear less healthy and energetic after just one or two nights of sleep deprivation.

Adequate "beauty sleep" improves skin hydration, leading to a smoother and firmer texture. Pores look smaller, and there are subtle changes in skin colour.

Skin also functions better with adequate sleep. The skin barrier is more resilient and recovers faster after injury and UV exposure. Inflammatory markers are decreased, and skin growth and renewal processes are improved. Sufficient sleep is also known to improve many skin disorders that involve inflammation, such as atopic dermatitis and psoriasis. Some studies have found that consistently high quality sleep can make people feel better about their appearance, and reduce signs of aging.

Why does my skin look different in the morning?

Your skin might look plumper and brighter immediately after waking. This is because gravity moves dermal fluid towards your legs when upright, whereas sleeping horizontally redistributes the fluid towards your face (though this can also accentuate eye bags).

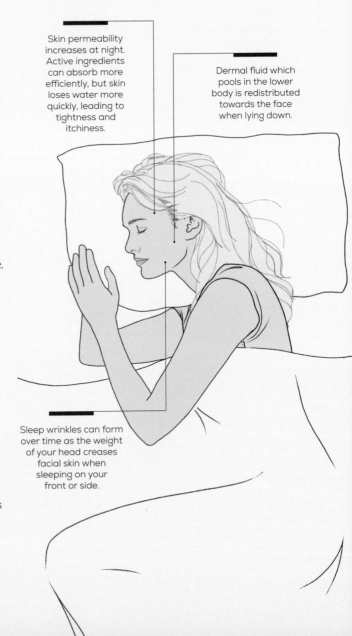

Skin permeability increases at night. Active ingredients can absorb more efficiently, but skin loses water more quickly, leading to tightness and itchiness.

Dermal fluid which pools in the lower body is redistributed towards the face when lying down.

Sleep wrinkles can form over time as the weight of your head creases facial skin when sleeping on your front or side.

How can I tell if a skincare product is really working?

Product labels and reviews can help you find products that are likely to work. But biology is complex, and products can be less effective for any one individual for many reasons. It can be difficult to tell if a product is actually causing a positive or negative change in your skin, or if it's unrelated.

Skin condition naturally fluctuates, and many other factors can explain changes. For example, a pimple that heals after you apply a treatment might have healed anyway (regression fallacy). Your skin might look better after you start using a cream after a summer holiday, but you also drastically reduced your sun exposure and drank less alcohol (confounding variables).

In addition, humans have many cognitive distortions that limit our ability to be objective. We interpret information according to our prior beliefs, so we're more likely to think a product works because the marketing was convincing (confirmation bias), or it would be a waste of money if it didn't (post-purchase rationalization). Plus we can be very confident about false memories. These biases are why well-controlled scientific experiments are performed. We can incorporate some principles of experimental design to get a better idea of whether products are working:

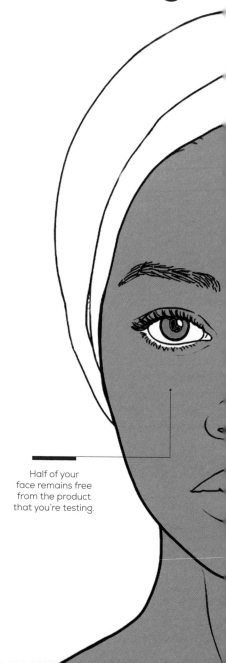

Half of your face remains free from the product that you're testing.

Half-face test

Apply a product to one side of the face, while leaving the other side untreated. Evaluate the product's performance by noting any differences between the two sides.

Introduce one new product at a time to your skincare routine. This limits the factors that may be affecting your skin, so any improvement or reaction is more likely to be caused by the product.

Try each product for two weeks or longer. This gives your skin time to adjust to the product. It also allows more time for natural fluctuations to occur, so you can rule out other potential causes. In general, the deeper the site of action, the longer it'll take to see changes. Ingredients that target collagen and deeper pigment can take over six months to have noticeable effects, while a moisturizer might work immediately.

Half-face test. Try a product on half your face only, so the other half can act as a comparison.

Cycle in and out. Try adding and removing a product from your routine to see if its use consistently matches changes in your skin.

Keep a skin record. This is useful for tracking changes in your skin, the products you're using, and any relevant lifestyle factors (food, menstrual cycle, exercise). This could include photos of your skin, which can help you see slow changes over time. Make sure you keep the lighting, camera angle, and brightness/contrast consistent.

Product applied to one side of the face.

Week 1 2 3 4 5 6 7 8 9 10

Cycling products in and out

Use a product consistently for a set amount of time, then take a break, and repeat. Record any changes in your skin.

Key

● *Use product*

● *No product*

How does diet affect my skin?

Food provides nutrients for your body, including your skin. A balanced diet rich in vegetables and healthy fats seems to be best for skin health.

Carbohydrates, fat, and protein provide energy for essential functions and are building blocks for skin. Some evidence suggests that that foods rich in the essential fatty acids omega-3 and omega-6, like flaxseed, evening primrose, and fish oils, can help with dry and inflammatory skin conditions.

However, there are many issues with diet and skin studies, which makes it difficult to draw strong conclusions.

Most interventional studies, where diet was changed and skin effects were tracked, involved college-aged males, which limits how applicable the results are to other demographics. Adding or removing one food from someone's usual diet can also change their other dietary preferences.

Observational studies often ask subjects to recall their food intake and skin condition, which is subject to self-editing and faulty recall. For example, the most highly cited study on dairy and acne asked women in their 30s and 40s what they ate when they were teenagers.

Even studies with potentially promising results are not necessarily helpful guidance. Big changes in diet can lead to unbalanced nutrition, disordered eating, and anxiety. Talk to your doctor before changing your diet significantly; in many cases, there are treatments with better success rates and fewer risks.

Diet and acne

Scientists have long noted lower rates of acne in non-Westernized populations, and the increase when they switched to Westernized lifestyles. Many studies have

It's difficult to conduct rigorous studies on diet and skin, so it's hard to point to any one culinary culprit that causes acne.

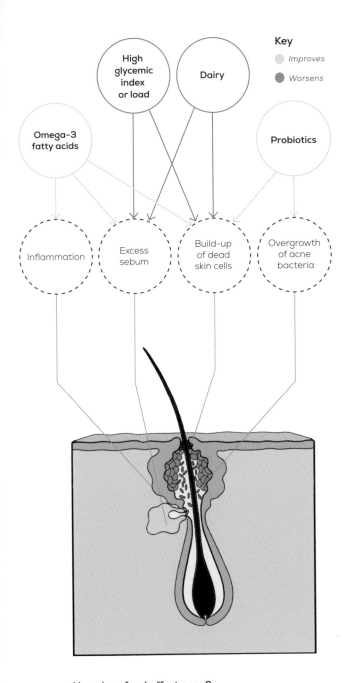

High glycemic index or load

Dairy

Omega-3 fatty acids

Probiotics

Inflammation

Excess sebum

Build-up of dead skin cells

Overgrowth of acne bacteria

VITAMINS AND SKIN

Many vitamins have important roles in normal skin function.

● **Vitamin A**, found in full-fat dairy, egg yolks, and plant pigments, is required for production and development of epidermal cells. Overconsumption of carotene-rich fruits and vegetables can turn skin orange.

● **Vitamin C** is the main water-soluble antioxidant in skin that protects against oxidative stress, and is needed for collagen production. It's in many fruits and vegetables.

● **Vitamin E** is the main oil-soluble antioxidant in skin that protects against oxidative stress. It is found in nuts, oils, and vegetables.

● **Vitamin B2 (riboflavin)** deficiency can lead to cracks at the corner of the mouth (angular cheilitis). Dairy and fortified grain products contain riboflavin.

● **Vitamin B3 (niacin)** is needed for the action of many skin enzymes. It's found in meat, fish, eggs, and grains.

● **Vitamin B7 (biotin)** is important for synthesizing keratin, which gives skin, hair, and nails much of their strength. It is found in egg yolks, legumes, and seeds.

How does food affect acne?

Some foods can potentially contribute to acne, while others may lead to improvements.

tried to identify specific dietary changes that may be contributing. The most evidence exists for diets high in refined sugar and carbohydrates that absorb quickly into blood (high glycemic index or load). There is also evidence that some dairy products may increase acne, including whey protein and milk. These are all thought to lead to increased pore clogging, sebum, and inflammation.

Despite these studies, the evidence is not strong enough to recommend dietary changes alone to manage acne.

Other skin effects

It's believed that a balanced diet rich in vegetables and essential fatty acids, and low in refined carbohydrates, saturated fats, and meat can mitigate some contributors to accelerated skin aging.

As well as providing many micronutrients, fruits and vegetables contain phytochemicals that could be beneficial to skin. Carotenoids and antioxidants like polyphenols can protect against sunlight and oxidative stress.

Some foods have reduced wrinkles in small studies, including raw almonds, mango, and cocoa. However, too much can have negative effects: while two cups of mango a week decreased wrinkles, six cups increased wrinkles, possibly due to high sugar levels.

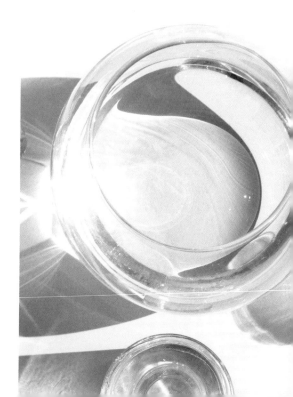

Drink water when you're thirsty. After that, more hydration won't make much of a difference.

Will drinking more water help my skin?

"Just drink more water" is popular advice for fixing virtually any skin problem. But there isn't much solid evidence to back it up.

The evidence indicates that drinking when you're thirsty will keep you adequately hydrated. Beyond that, drinking additional water doesn't seem to make much of a difference, since your body has many mechanisms for maintaining its water balance. When thirst might not be enough of a guide, like during intense exercise or hot weather, it can be helpful to consciously drink more water.

There are a few studies on the effects of drinking extra water on skin. The results weren't very impressive: some people's skin hydration and smoothness increased, but it seemed to require drinking an extra 2 litres (8 cups) of water a day on top of normal consumption, and improvements were more likely for people who didn't drink much water to begin with (less than 1 litre, or 4 cups). The skin changes were comparable to using a good moisturizer.

Anecdotally, many people report changes in their skin when they drink more water, but it's difficult to differentiate this from the many other factors that could've affected their skin at the same time.

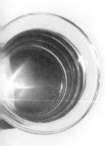

AM I CONSUMING ENOUGH WATER?

Staying hydrated is easier than you might think.

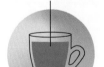

99% water

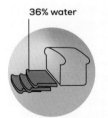

36% water

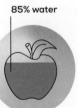

85% water

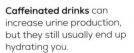

Caffeinated drinks can increase urine production, but they still usually end up hydrating you.

Solid food provides around 20% of our daily water intake. Even dry foods like bread contain a lot of water!

Why am I having an allergic reaction?

Allergies are overreactions to harmless substances (allergens) by the immune system. Many allergies affect skin since it is in constant contact with the environment.

Skin allergies

Allergic contact dermatitis is the most common type of skin allergy. This is a delayed type IV hypersensitivity reaction, where white blood cells respond to an allergen on your skin by triggering a chain reaction. A day or two after exposure, the area turns red and itchy, and may crack or blister.

Many substances we encounter daily can be contact allergens for some people. Whether your immune system becomes sensitized to a particular substance depends on many factors including genetics, skin condition, the substance's properties, the quantity involved, and frequency of contact. It can take years of exposure before sensitization occurs. It's estimated that up to 20% of people have a contact allergy.

Once you develop an allergy to a substance, it will trigger a reaction if enough is detected by your immune system.

It can be difficult to identify the specific substance causing a reaction, because your skin encounters many substances

COMMON SKIN ALLERGENS

These common skin allergens may cause redness, itching, rashes, and swelling as your immune system goes into overdrive.

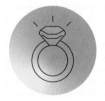

Nickel
One of the most common contact allergens. Often found in earrings, necklaces, watches, buttons, and zips.

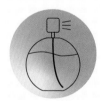

Fragrance
Reactions can occur with perfume or fragranced personal care and household products.

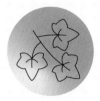

Poison ivy
Causes rashes, along with other *Toxicodendron* species that produce urushiol.

every day. Allergy clinics can perform patch tests with common allergens. If you react to cosmetic products, you may find it useful to look at the ingredients in all the products you use. Keep in mind that cosmetic allergens can also be found in cleaning products, detergents, fabrics, air fresheners, paints, and glues.

You should avoid any substances you've developed an allergy to. Allergy symptoms can be reduced with topical steroids. Supporting your skin barrier can also reduce the chance of allergic reactions.

Other allergies

Other types of allergies can provoke a reaction on the skin. These are usually immediate type I hypersensitivity reactions, and include food, pet, and pollen allergies. Skin contact with food can increase the chance of developing food allergies, particularly if skin is broken and inflamed. Research has found that managing eczema

well can reduce the chance of food allergies by improving skin barrier function.
If you're allergic to a particular food, you might also be allergic to it in your beauty products. Food allergens are generally proteins, which may still be present in minimally refined cosmetic ingredients. Sprays and shower products are higher risk as any allergens are more likely to be inhaled and impair breathing.

Botanical ingredients are listed by their Latin names, so make sure you're familiar with the Latin name of anything you're allergic to.

Flowers
Many plants can be contact allergens, including primroses, daffodils, grevilleas, and sunflowers.

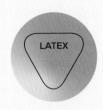

Latex
Allergens are usually ingredients used in processing latex, or proteins from the latex tree.

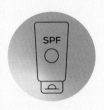

Sunscreen
Some sunscreen ingredients cause allergic reactions only after exposure to UV (photoallergy).

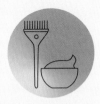

Permanent hair dye
Contains p-phenylenediamine (PPD) and related substances.

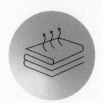

Fabrics and leather
Formaldehyde resins and dimethyl fumarate used in leather tanning are common culprits.

Do DIY skincare recipes work?

There are lots of recipes for homemade skincare online, but most aren't safe and effective.

While some beneficial ingredients are found in household items, they are not optimized for delivery into skin and the concentrations are usually too low to be effective:

- Yoghurt contains lactic acid at below 1% (5–10% in skincare)
- Lemon juice contains 0.04% vitamin C and 0.0001% vitamin B3 (5–15% and 2–10% in skincare, respectively)
- Coffee beans contain 1–2% caffeine (7% caffeine gel used to reduce appearance of cellulite)

Safety

The biggest risks with DIY skincare are irritation, rashes, and infection from microbial spoilage, as recipes rarely include effective preservatives.

Common DIY ingredients like essential oils, fruit, and spices are irritating to skin when used in high concentrations or left on skin. Some ingredients carry extra risks:

Citrus oils and juices often contain psoralens, which cause blistering burns with sun exposure (phytophotodermatitis).
Lemon juice has been reported to permanently damage melanin-producing cells, leading to uneven, permanently bleached patches of skin.
Apple cider vinegar can cause burns and scarring due to its high acidity, especially if applied for prolonged periods or covered with bandages.

DIY sunscreen recipes give poor and inconsistent sun protection. Most recipes use zinc oxide, which clumps easily, and kitchen tools can't achieve the particle distribution required for UV protection.

Some safe DIY recipes

Bath bombs – mix baking soda, citric acid, and cornflour.
Lip balms – mix molten beeswax, oils, and vitamin E.
Whipped body butters – whip melted butters and oils together.
Fresh face masks – can be applied for 5–10 minutes then washed off:

- Oatmeal: moisturizing, contains soothing avenanthramides.
- Kiwifruit, papaya, pumpkin: contain exfoliating enzymes.
- Green tea: contains soothing antioxidants.
- Yoghurt, honey, plant oils: moisturizing.

Face scrubs – mix sugar, salt, or rice powder with water or cleanser immediately before use.

Advanced DIY skincare

More advanced DIY formulations using cosmetic-grade ingredients can be safe and effective, and makes for a fun hobby. You can follow recipes created by experienced formulators, or take a formulation course.

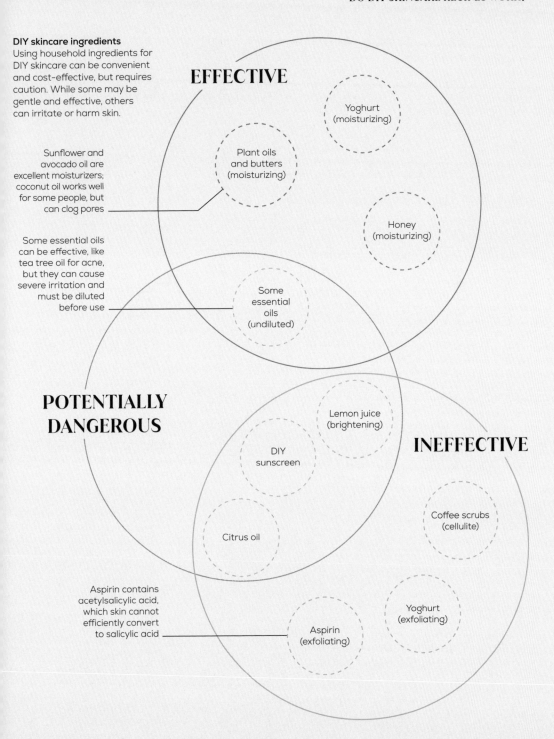

DIY skincare ingredients
Using household ingredients for DIY skincare can be convenient and cost-effective, but requires caution. While some may be gentle and effective, others can irritate or harm skin.

Sunflower and avocado oil are excellent moisturizers; coconut oil works well for some people, but can clog pores

Some essential oils can be effective, like tea tree oil for acne, but they can cause severe irritation and must be diluted before use

Aspirin contains acetylsalicylic acid, which skin cannot efficiently convert to salicylic acid

EFFECTIVE

POTENTIALLY DANGEROUS

INEFFECTIVE

Yoghurt (moisturizing)

Plant oils and butters (moisturizing)

Honey (moisturizing)

Some essential oils (undiluted)

Lemon juice (brightening)

DIY sunscreen

Citrus oil

Coffee scrubs (cellulite)

Aspirin (exfoliating)

Yoghurt (exfoliating)

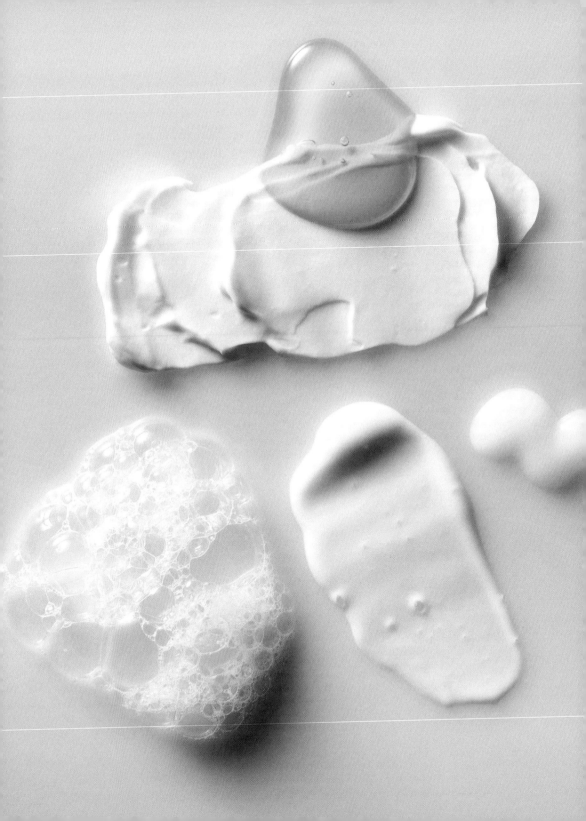

The biggest risks
with DIY skincare
are irritation, rashes,
and infection from
microbial spoilage, as
recipes rarely include
effective preservatives.

Why do I need to wear sunscreen?

Sunscreens reduce the amount of UV that reaches your skin. Only 3% of sunlight at ground level is UV, but individual UV photons are highly energetic – it's the main external cause of skin damage.

Two types of UV from the sun can harm our skin:
- **UVA** (315–400 nm): longer, lower-energy wavelengths that mostly damage skin by creating reactive free radicals. UVA can penetrate deeper into skin, damaging dermal collagen and elastin.
- **UVB** (280–315 nm): shorter, more energetic wavelengths that directly damage DNA. It is strongly linked to sunburn and skin cancer.

Both types contribute to tanning, cumulative skin damage, premature skin aging, uneven pigmentation, and immune suppression, which increases the risk of cancer.

The rise in recreational sun exposure in recent decades, coupled with a thinner ozone layer, has resulted in increased UV exposure, meaning that sun protection is more important than ever.

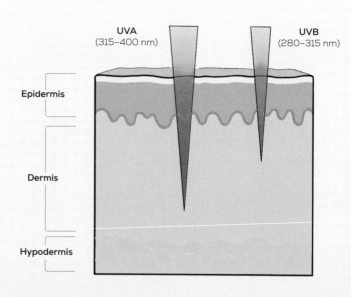

UVA
(315–400 nm)

UVB
(280–315 nm)

Epidermis

Dermis

Hypodermis

UV and skin
The sun's UVA and UVB rays penetrate to different depths in unprotected skin.

WHEN TO WEAR SUNSCREEN

While excessive UV exposure is harmful, some sun exposure is beneficial, such as for vitamin D synthesis. These guidelines have been developed by Australian health organizations to balance skin cancer risk and health benefits, for skin with different UV sensitivity.

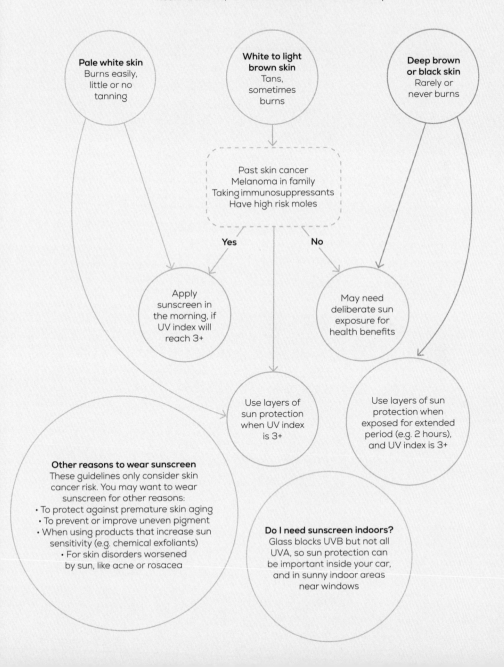

Pale white skin
Burns easily, little or no tanning

White to light brown skin
Tans, sometimes burns

Deep brown or black skin
Rarely or never burns

Past skin cancer
Melanoma in family
Taking immunosuppressants
Have high risk moles

Yes

No

Apply sunscreen in the morning, if UV index will reach 3+

May need deliberate sun exposure for health benefits

Use layers of sun protection when UV index is 3+

Use layers of sun protection when exposed for extended period (e.g. 2 hours), and UV index is 3+

Other reasons to wear sunscreen
These guidelines only consider skin cancer risk. You may want to wear sunscreen for other reasons:
• To protect against premature skin aging
• To prevent or improve uneven pigment
• When using products that increase sun sensitivity (e.g. chemical exfoliants)
• For skin disorders worsened by sun, like acne or rosacea

Do I need sunscreen indoors?
Glass blocks UVB but not all UVA, so sun protection can be important inside your car, and in sunny indoor areas near windows

Do I need sun protection if I have darker skin?

Melanin is a natural sunscreen, but it often doesn't provide enough protection.

Skin colour

Skin colour reflects the types, amount, and distribution of melanin. Two types of melanin (eumelanin and pheomelanin) are present in all skin tones, but are more abundant in darker skin.

Brown-black eumelanin absorbs a broad spectrum of UV, and buffers against oxidative damage. In contrast, yellow-red pheomelanin produces free radicals in UVA, and is thought to increase sun damage.

The tanning response is largely determined by genetics, and involves multiple processes initiated by sunlight. Melanin immediately darkens and its distribution changes in UVA, and this effect lasts for around a day. UVB (and some UVA) causes delayed tanning, where new melanin appears a few days later. In darker skin, high energy blue-violet light can increase pigment, which takes longer to fade. The stratum corneum thickens with UV exposure, and provides over half the sun protection in lighter skin.

Dark skin

Melanin protects against many forms of skin damage including sunburn, cancer, and some types of photoaging. Very dark skin can have in-built protection equivalent to SPF 15. However, dark skin can still burn,

HOW MUCH PROTECTION?

Darker skin can be more resistant to sun damage, but looks can be deceiving.

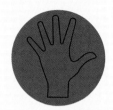

Dark skin tones
Melanin in naturally dark skin can provide up to SPF 15 protection, depending on skin tone.

White skin
White people in the US are 70 times more likely to develop skin cancer than Black people.

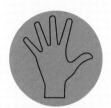

Suntan
UVA and UVB from the sun can increase melanin, but only gives an estimated protection of SPF 1–4.

so sun protective measures are still recommended. In a 2016 survey, 13.2% of Black people, 29.7% of Hispanic people and 42.5% of white people reported sunburn in the previous year.

Skin cancer risk is strongly linked to melanin. Some non-white people also have other mechanisms that reduce skin cancer risk, such as more efficient DNA repair and destruction of abnormal cells. While skin cancer incidence is closely related to sun exposure in white skin, the link is far weaker for non-white groups (but also less studied).

However, sun exposure isn't the only contributor to skin cancer. Skin cancers often appear in areas that don't receive sunlight, and people with darker skin tend to have poorer outcomes due to later detection. If you have darker skin, you might not need to worry as much about sun protection, but you should monitor unusual skin marks more closely, and seek prompt medical attention.

Melanin also protects against some forms of premature sun-induced skin aging. UV damage to dermal proteins leads to wrinkles, which show up decades later in non-white skin.

On the other hand, non-white skin is more prone to pigment changes and disorders that are exacerbated by many wavelengths in sunlight. Look for a sunscreen with high UVA protection, and use tinted products containing iron oxides for visible light protection.

Tanning

It's tempting to think a "base tan" can protect against further sun damage. Unfortunately, a suntan only gives the equivalent of SPF 1–4. Sunless tanners also provide only SPF 3–4 (but with much less damage). Tans from sunbeds have been measured to give very poor protection (below SPF 1.5), since they use more UVA. They increase melanoma risk by 75% if used before age 35.

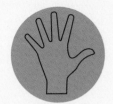

Sunbed tan
UVA-induced indoor tanning gives less than SPF 1.5 protection, after more than ten tanning sessions.

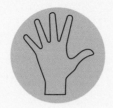

Sunscreen
Commercial sunscreens usually provide SPF 15–50+ protection, if applied correctly.

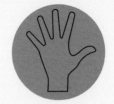

Fake tan
Artificial tanning products create a brown layer on skin, which gives SPF 3–4 protection.

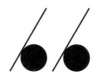

Higher protection
is achieved when
the filters are spread
on skin as evenly as
possible, with minimal
gaps where UV can
get through.

What kinds of sunscreen are there?

Sunscreens contain active ingredients (UV filters) that absorb incoming UV and convert it into harmless forms of energy, like heat.

UV filters are divided into two categories. **Organic "chemical" filters** have carbon-based structures that can absorb UV. **Inorganic "mineral" or "physical" filters** are solid particles of zinc oxide or titanium dioxide. Contrary to popular belief, these ingredients do not work by reflecting UV, but also mostly absorb UV. Particle size is crucial to how efficiently they work, as well as the wavelengths absorbed. Solid UV filters also scatter a small amount of UV (less than 10%). This includes inorganic filters as well as some organic ones, like bisoctrizole.

In addition to the active ingredients, the overall formulation will influence how much protection a sunscreen gives. Higher protection is achieved when the filters are spread on skin as evenly as possible, so there are minimal gaps where UV can get through.

Visible light protection

Most sunscreens offer little protection against high energy blue-violet wavelengths of visible light from the sun, which have recently been found to darken pigment in darker skin. However, iron oxide pigments in tinted products like foundations and tinted sunscreen will protect against visible light, although no protection standard like SPF exists for easy comparison between products.

DIFFERENT TYPES OF SUNSCREEN INGREDIENTS

There are two major categories of UV filters used in sunscreens, but there are more similarities than differences in how they work.

Organic filters
Most organic filters work by absorbing UV before it reaches the skin, and converting it to a tiny amount of heat.

Inorganic filters
Inorganic (and some organic) sunscreens also work primarily by absorbing UV, but a small amount of UV (5–10%) is reflected or scattered.

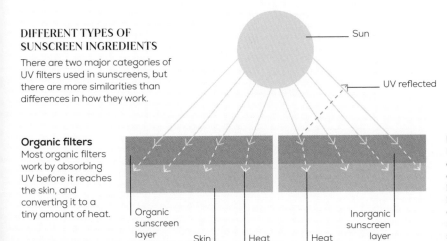

Sun

UV reflected

Organic sunscreen layer

Skin

Heat

Heat

Inorganic sunscreen layer

How do I choose a sunscreen?

A sunscreen should be protective enough for the activities you're doing. It should also be comfortable and budget-friendly, so it can be generously applied and reapplied.

Protection level

Some protection claims on sunscreen labels are standardized:

Sun Protection Factor (SPF) is the main metric used worldwide to compare different sunscreens. It measures the protection a sunscreen gives against UV-induced reddening (erythema) compared to bare skin. For example, a properly applied layer of SPF 30 sunscreen should allow skin to receive 30 times more UV before burning. SPF is designed to be proportional to protection: SPF 15 will let in twice as much burning UV (6.7%) as SPF 30 (3.3%), so it gives half the protection. SPF is currently measured using human volunteers, following a strict protocol. Two milligrams of sunscreen are evenly applied per square centimetre of skin, before exposing it to bursts of UV from a special lamp. Skin reddening is mostly (80–90%) caused by UVB with some contribution from UVA, so SPF primarily reflects UVB protection.

UVA protection ratings differ by region:

- **"Broad spectrum" or UVA circle logo** This means the UVA protection is proportional to SPF. In most regions this means the UVAPF is at least one-third of the SPF, and 10% of the UV protection is for wavelengths longer than 370 nm (critical wavelength). In the US, only the critical wavelength requirement is needed.
- **Persistent Pigment Darkening (PPD)** Like SPF, this is tested using human volunteers. It measures the protection a sunscreen gives against UVA-induced persistent pigment darkening, compared to bare skin.
- **PA** This is commonly used in Asia and converts PPD to a range: PA+ = PPD 2–4, PA++ = PPD 4–8, PA+++ = PPD 8–16, PA++++ = PPD 16+

For daily wear, a broad spectrum sunscreen with SPF 30 or higher is recommended.

Water resistance To measure water resistance, SPF is tested after immersion in water for a set period, and compared to the original SPF. The drop in SPF allowed for a water-resistant sunscreen differs around the world. For example, US and Australian water-resistant sunscreens provide the labelled SPF after immersion, while the EU allows SPF to drop by half.

Water-resistant sunscreens are usually also more resistant to sand, rubbing, and movement, so they tend to be better suited for outdoor activities.

Comfort and budget

The level of protection depends heavily on application. The quantity is most important – to get the labelled SPF, you need to apply the same amount as in SPF testing (see right).

Studies have found that most people only apply 25–50% of the recommended amount. SPF is roughly proportional to the amount applied, so many people are getting only SPF 7.5 from an SPF 30 sunscreen! Hence a lot of innovation has gone towards creating lightweight sunscreens that are more comfortable to apply.

Chemical or physical?

In practice, the main difference between chemical (organic) and physical (inorganic) sunscreens is texture. Chemical sunscreens tend to be lighter and can sometimes be greasy, while physical sunscreens are usually heavier and more drying. Additionally, some people find specific chemical filters irritating to the skin and eyes, while physical filters often look white on darker skin (tinted sunscreens can make this less noticeable). Combination or hybrid sunscreens contain both types of filters.

Studies have found that most people only apply 25–50% of the recommended amount of sunscreen.

HOW TO APPLY SUNSCREEN

Regardless of what SPF you use, you won't get adequate protection if you apply it incorrectly.

How much? ¼ teaspoon (1.25 ml) or two generous finger lengths for the face, one shot glass (35 ml) for an average adult body, with roughly 1 teaspoon (5 ml) for each of the following: face, neck, and ears; each limb; front of body; back.

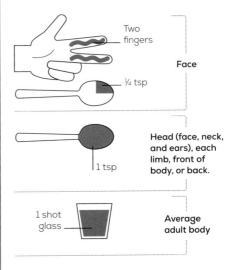

Two fingers

Face

¼ tsp

1 tsp

Head (face, neck, and ears), each limb, front of body, or back.

1 shot glass

Average adult body

When? Before sun exposure – allow 5–10 minutes for sunscreen to dry and settle. Sunscreen should be reapplied every two hours as the sunscreen layer shifts over time and leaves gaps. Also reapply after swimming and towelling.

With other products? Sunscreen works best when the layer is disturbed as little as possible. When layering, it goes after your other skincare products and before makeup. Sunscreen does not need to be absorbed into skin to "activate". It should not be mixed with other products as this can create gaps in the protective layer.

How? Spread sunscreen evenly over skin. Avoid vigorous rubbing, which can reduce protection.

Can sunscreen be bad for me?

There is no compelling evidence of long-term health harms from sunscreen, despite over 50 years of widespread use.

In contrast, there is very good evidence for the need to protect against excessive sun exposure. Sunscreen is a therapeutic product in many countries, so their ingredients are some of the most closely regulated and scrutinized in skincare (see p12).

From time to time, anxiety-inducing news stories have questioned potential risks associated with wearing sunscreen. The most common concerns revolve around vitamin D deficiency and ingredient safety.

Studies have failed to find a link between sunscreen use and reduced vitamin D.

Vitamin D deficiency
UVB causes sunburn, skin cancer, and photoaging, but it also helps convert 7-dehydrocholesterol to vitamin D in the skin. Since sunscreen blocks UVB, there's long been speculation that sunscreen could reduce vitamin D, which has important roles in bone and metabolic health, and immune function. However, studies have failed to find a link between reduced vitamin D and sunscreen use, although it is linked to staying indoors and protective clothing. This is likely because people only use sunscreen when going into the sun, sunscreen is never applied sufficiently to block all UV, and not much UVB is needed for adequate vitamin D.

Following sun exposure guidelines (see p85) will ensure adequate vitamin D for most people. If vitamin D is still low, eating more vitamin D-rich foods and taking a supplement are usually recommended over increasing sun exposure.

Endocrine (hormone) disruption
Chemical sunscreens (see p89) are often said to be endocrine disruptors. While some chemical sunscreens have had hormonal effects in cell and animal studies, these typically use unrealistically high doses. Current evidence indicates that the exposure from normal sunscreen use is

hundreds to thousands of times too low to cause harm. The ingredients of most concern have been used for decades without evidence of widespread impacts.

Additionally, there are around 20 chemical sunscreen ingredients in common use, many of which do not have any known endocrine effects. Newer chemical sunscreens are designed to be inherently less risky, with structures that cannot normally pass through skin.

Nanoparticles

Zinc oxide and titanium dioxide are used in sunscreens as solid particles. Nanoparticles (particles 1–100 nanometres wide) give better UV protection with less white cast on skin. There has been concern that these could absorb through skin and cause harm, but they do not seem to penetrate past the upper stratum corneum. However, large amounts inhaled from spray sunscreens can be hazardous.

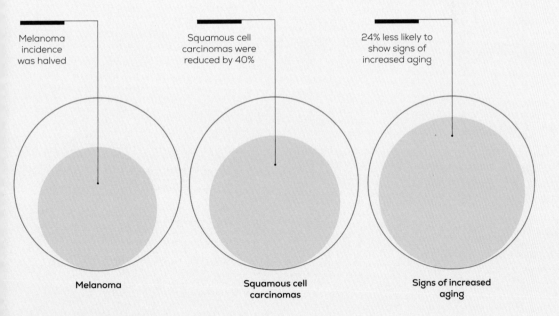

Melanoma incidence was halved

Squamous cell carcinomas were reduced by 40%

24% less likely to show signs of increased aging

Melanoma

Squamous cell carcinomas

Signs of increased aging

The importance of sunscreen

The largest clinical trial on sunscreen use was conducted in Queensland, Australia from 1992 to 1996. For 4.5 years, participants applied sunscreen either daily or when they normally would, and the results between the two groups were compared.

Key

◯ Normal sunscreen users

⬤ Daily sunscreen users

How else can I protect my skin from the sun?

While sunscreen is useful, layering multiple forms of sun protection is the most effective strategy.

This way, shortcomings in one protective layer can be covered by another.

Avoiding high UV exposure

UV is highest in summer, between 10am and 4pm. Look up the UV index for your specific time and location.

Sun protective clothing

UV-protective clothing has many advantages. Regular reapplication isn't necessary, it's harder to miss spots or underapply, and it protects against all wavelengths. Some clothes have a labelled ultraviolet protection factor (UPF), calculated similarly to SPF. Protection from clothes with no UPF rating is less predictable. Intensely coloured, tightly knitted synthetics tend to protect best. A white cotton t-shirt is typically only UPF 5–9. Polyester offers 3–4 times more protection than cotton. Unfortunately, more protective fabrics are less comfortable in hot weather – in one survey, one-third of summer clothes had below UPF 15.

THE UV INDEX

The UV index is an international code that gauges the risk of sunburn. Higher numbers indicate stronger UV, and greater need to take sun protective measures.

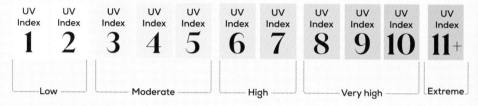

UV Index **1**	UV Index **2**	UV Index **3**	UV Index **4**	UV Index **5**	UV Index **6**	UV Index **7**	UV Index **8**	UV Index **9**	UV Index **10**	UV Index **11+**
Low		Moderate			High		Very high			Extreme

Exposure category

Shade

Shade is useful for protecting against direct sunlight. However, much of our UV exposure is indirect, which is why you can still get sunburnt in the shade. The indirect UV you receive is roughly proportional to the amount of sky you can see, so a building that blocks out a lot of sky gives much more protection than a beach umbrella, for example. Most ground surfaces – including water, concrete, and sand – reflect below 10% UV. Some reflect substantially more, including snow (up to 90%) and dry beach sand (4–30%).

Hats

Hats made of thick material will block direct sunlight, but give limited protection against indirect UV as not much sky is blocked, particularly for the lower face. Broad-brimmed hats with flaps are more protective. A flat-brimmed cowboy hat is estimated to reduce facial UV exposure by 2–6 times.

Sunglasses

Skin cancer and photoaging commonly occur around the eyes. Large close-fitting sunglasses block more UV, and can protect against sun-induced vision problems and cataracts.

Dietary supplements

Niacinamide has been found to reduce non-melanoma skin cancers in high-risk patients, and some antioxidants might reduce sunburn, but the benefits of sun-protective supplements are not well substantiated. They should not be considered substitutes for limiting the UV that reaches the skin in the first place.

Skincare ingredients

Iron oxides in skin-coloured products can protect against blue light, which can darken pigment. Vitamins C and E have been found to reduce sunburn. Niacinamide can potentially reduce skin cancer risk.

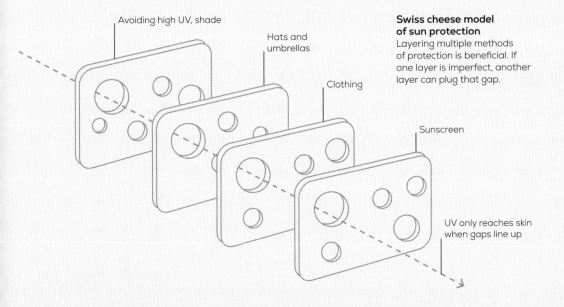

Avoiding high UV, shade

Hats and umbrellas

Clothing

Swiss cheese model of sun protection
Layering multiple methods of protection is beneficial. If one layer is imperfect, another layer can plug that gap.

Sunscreen

UV only reaches skin when gaps line up

Skincare specifics

What's going on with my skin?

Many conditions can affect our skin, ranging from mild irritations to severe outbreaks.

Some disappear spontaneously or with care and treatment, while others are lifelong conditions that can be managed to reduce discomfort or prevent complications.

Pharmacists can usually provide advice and recommend over-the-counter treatments. However, many skin conditions present in similar ways, so it's important to seek an accurate diagnosis from a doctor if there is no improvement. You should also seek medical advice if there is scarring, or if the condition is affecting your mental health.

It can be helpful to book a consultation with a skincare professional if you're uncertain about whether your skincare products are appropriate for your skin.

WHAT IS ROSACEA?

Rosacea is an inflammatory condition that causes flushing, visible blood vessels, and pimple-like bumps. It's thought to be caused by a combination of environmental and genetic factors. The face is particularly susceptible due to its sensitivity and high concentration of blood vessels.

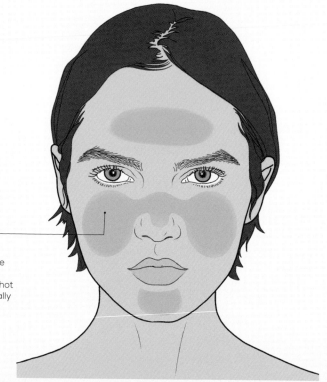

Rosacea regions
Rosacea shows up on the cheeks, nose, chin, and forehead. Triggers include hot food, sun, and heat. Typically develops after age 30.

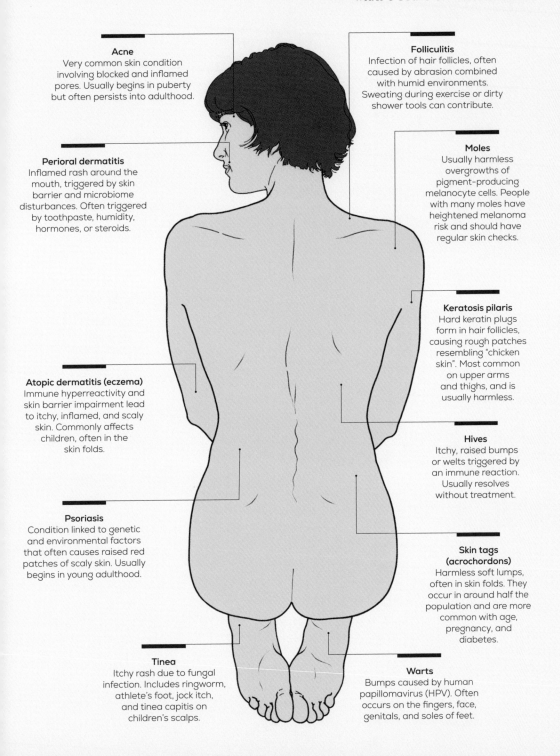

WHAT'S GOING ON WITH MY SKIN?

Acne
Very common skin condition involving blocked and inflamed pores. Usually begins in puberty but often persists into adulthood.

Folliculitis
Infection of hair follicles, often caused by abrasion combined with humid environments. Sweating during exercise or dirty shower tools can contribute.

Perioral dermatitis
Inflamed rash around the mouth, triggered by skin barrier and microbiome disturbances. Often triggered by toothpaste, humidity, hormones, or steroids.

Moles
Usually harmless overgrowths of pigment-producing melanocyte cells. People with many moles have heightened melanoma risk and should have regular skin checks.

Atopic dermatitis (eczema)
Immune hyperreactivity and skin barrier impairment lead to itchy, inflamed, and scaly skin. Commonly affects children, often in the skin folds.

Keratosis pilaris
Hard keratin plugs form in hair follicles, causing rough patches resembling "chicken skin". Most common on upper arms and thighs, and is usually harmless.

Hives
Itchy, raised bumps or welts triggered by an immune reaction. Usually resolves without treatment.

Psoriasis
Condition linked to genetic and environmental factors that often causes raised red patches of scaly skin. Usually begins in young adulthood.

Skin tags (acrochordons)
Harmless soft lumps, often in skin folds. They occur in around half the population and are more common with age, pregnancy, and diabetes.

Tinea
Itchy rash due to fungal infection. Includes ringworm, athlete's foot, jock itch, and tinea capitis on children's scalps.

Warts
Bumps caused by human papillomavirus (HPV). Often occurs on the fingers, face, genitals, and soles of feet.

How do skincare products get ingredients into my skin?

How deep a skincare ingredient ends up in the skin depends on its inherent properties, as well as product formulation and application method.

The chemical properties of an ingredient determine how it interacts with skin. Ingredients that tend to get past the stratum corneum are small (molecular weight below 500 daltons) and have a moderate polarity (balance of charge, which determines solubility in water and oil). This means that a potentially beneficial ingredient might not be able to reach the part of the skin where it could work. However, many techniques can improve delivery into skin.

Derivatives

An ingredient's structure can be chemically altered to improve its properties. The new version is called a derivative.

Derivatives are often designed to penetrate deeper into the skin. They can also be more stable, leading to longer product shelf lives and less decomposition after applying. Vitamin A and C derivatives are often used in skincare for this reason.

Some derivatives have similar biological activities to the original ingredient, but many are inactive and must be activated in the skin. Evidence for this activation is often limited.

Formulation

Many aspects of product formulation control skin penetration. Some ingredients are delivered more effectively by particular formula types, like gels versus creams. Formulation pH can dramatically change absorption.

How well a formula delivers an ingredient into skin is difficult to predict accurately, and optimization can be a long process – this is a large part of why formulas cannot be judged by their ingredient lists alone.

Special delivery systems can also help ingredients absorb. For example, encapsulation techniques enclose the ingredient with a protective barrier. These can help the ingredient adhere to skin, or act as a shuttle to transport it into skin. Encapsulation can also improve stability or allow slow release, which reduces irritation.

Application methods

Some application methods can increase skin permeability, or push ingredients deeper. Hydrated skin is more permeable to many substances. Products can be applied to wet skin, or a hydrating product can be applied immediately before or after an active.

Occlusive skin coverings that trap water can also increase hydration, such as acne patches and sheet masks.

INCREASING PENETRATION OF VITAMIN C

L-Ascorbic acid (vitamin C) has many skin benefits but does not absorb into skin efficiently. These techniques can help increase penetration into the skin.

Encapsulation

Many materials are used to encapsulate ascorbic acid in skincare products to improve penetration and stability, including liposomes.

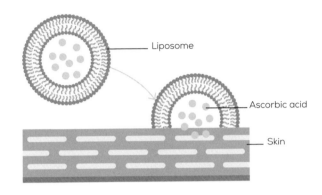

Liposome

Ascorbic acid

Skin

Derivatives

A short carbon chain can be added to make 3-O-ethyl ascorbic acid, which has less charge and hence greater absorption. Ascorbic acid is released after absorption.

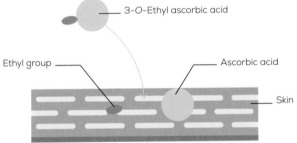

3-O-Ethyl ascorbic acid

Ethyl group

Ascorbic acid

Skin

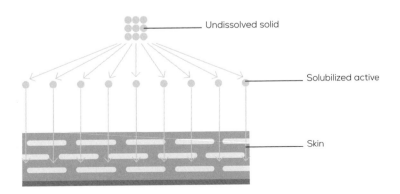

Undissolved solid

Solubilized active

Skin

Solvents and surfactants

Solvents and surfactants aid delivery by keeping ingredients dissolved.

What can skincare products do compared with clinical treatments?

Skincare products and clinical treatments are complementary approaches, rather than separate alternatives.

Our skin is an excellent barrier, which has been crucial for our survival. However, this same barrier makes it difficult for certain skincare treatments to penetrate. Clinical treatments can be useful for deeper skin concerns, and more substantial or rapid changes. However, skincare products are still important for maintaining these results.

Skincare (topical) products

Skincare is applied to the skin's surface, so the concentration of ingredients will generally be highest at the top, forming a gradient as we go deeper into the skin.

As a result, skincare products tend to work most effectively at the top of the skin. They are particularly useful for maintaining the skin's condition, and protecting it from environmental insults. Products like moisturizers, cleansers, sunscreens, and chemical exfoliants don't need to penetrate beyond the stratum corneum. Skincare products are also very useful for treating problems close to the skin's surface like acne, irritation, and infections. Some can target deeper concerns, like texture and pigment, but require months of consistent use for noticeable changes.

Clinical treatments

Cosmetic treatments performed by professionals are useful for targeting the deeper concerns that skincare products can't effectively reach, and for changing underlying muscle and fat. They can also deliver faster and more dramatic results.

However, there is a higher risk of side effects. The results are also often very dependent on the practitioner and how you communicate with them. When choosing a practitioner, look at examples of their work that resemble what you want, and make sure you understand the potential side effects. For example, if you have darker skin, it's a good idea to seek a practitioner with experience treating similar skin tones to yours, since post-inflammatory hyperpigmentation is a common side effect. It's also important to check for qualifications and accreditations. Treatments performed by unqualified practitioners can be extremely risky, and cause life-threatening complications or permanent disfigurement.

Examples of clinical treatments

Chemical peels create controlled injury to the skin to trigger its repair processes. They also help loosen the top layers of skin, although they don't necessarily cause visible peeling. They can be performed at different depths. Many peels use the same ingredients found in cosmetics like hydroxy acids and tretinoin, but at higher concentrations.

Dermabrasion and microdermabrasion mechanically remove the top layers of skin, like a deep version of physical exfoliation.
Ultrasound and radiofrequency treatments deliver heat into the skin to induce collagen production and give a "skin tightening" effect.
Laser and intense pulsed light (IPL) treatments use intense light to selectively destroy components of the skin (see pp125–127).
LED devices use light to stimulate different biological responses, depending on the wavelengths used. They can reduce inflammation, stimulate collagen, reduce acne bacteria, or speed up healing.
Botox is used to freeze muscles, usually for reducing wrinkles (see pp104–105).
Fillers are gel-like substances injected to add volume, commonly to the cheeks and lips. They are mostly broken down by the body over six months to two years. Filler materials include hyaluronic acid, calcium hydroxyapatite, and polylactic acid.
Deoxycholic acid injections are used to dissolve fat. For example, they can be used to reduce fat in the neck area.
Thread lifting uses dissolvable medical threads to pull the skin upwards.

Platelet rich plasma (PRP) treatments involve taking some of your blood, separating out the platelets, and injecting them back into the skin to induce healing responses.
Microneedling treatments puncture the skin with tiny needles. Shorter needles create channels for topical products to penetrate deeper, while longer needles cause controlled wounding to stimulate collagen and even out texture. It can be combined with radiofrequency, which increases the response by adding heat.

How deep do things go?
Skincare products can be effective at targeting issues in the upper layers of the skin, whereas clinical treatments can have more dramatic results, reaching into deeper layers of skin.

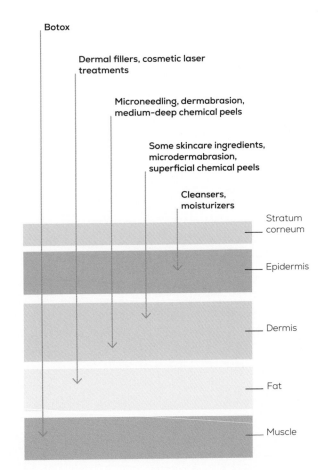

Botox

Dermal fillers, cosmetic laser treatments

Microneedling, dermabrasion, medium-deep chemical peels

Some skincare ingredients, microdermabrasion, superficial chemical peels

Cleansers, moisturizers

Stratum corneum

Epidermis

Dermis

Fat

Muscle

Where is botox injected?

Botox is used to soften dynamic wrinkles, such as frown lines, crow's feet, and lip lines. It can also be used to raise the eyebrows to provide a subtle non-surgical lift.

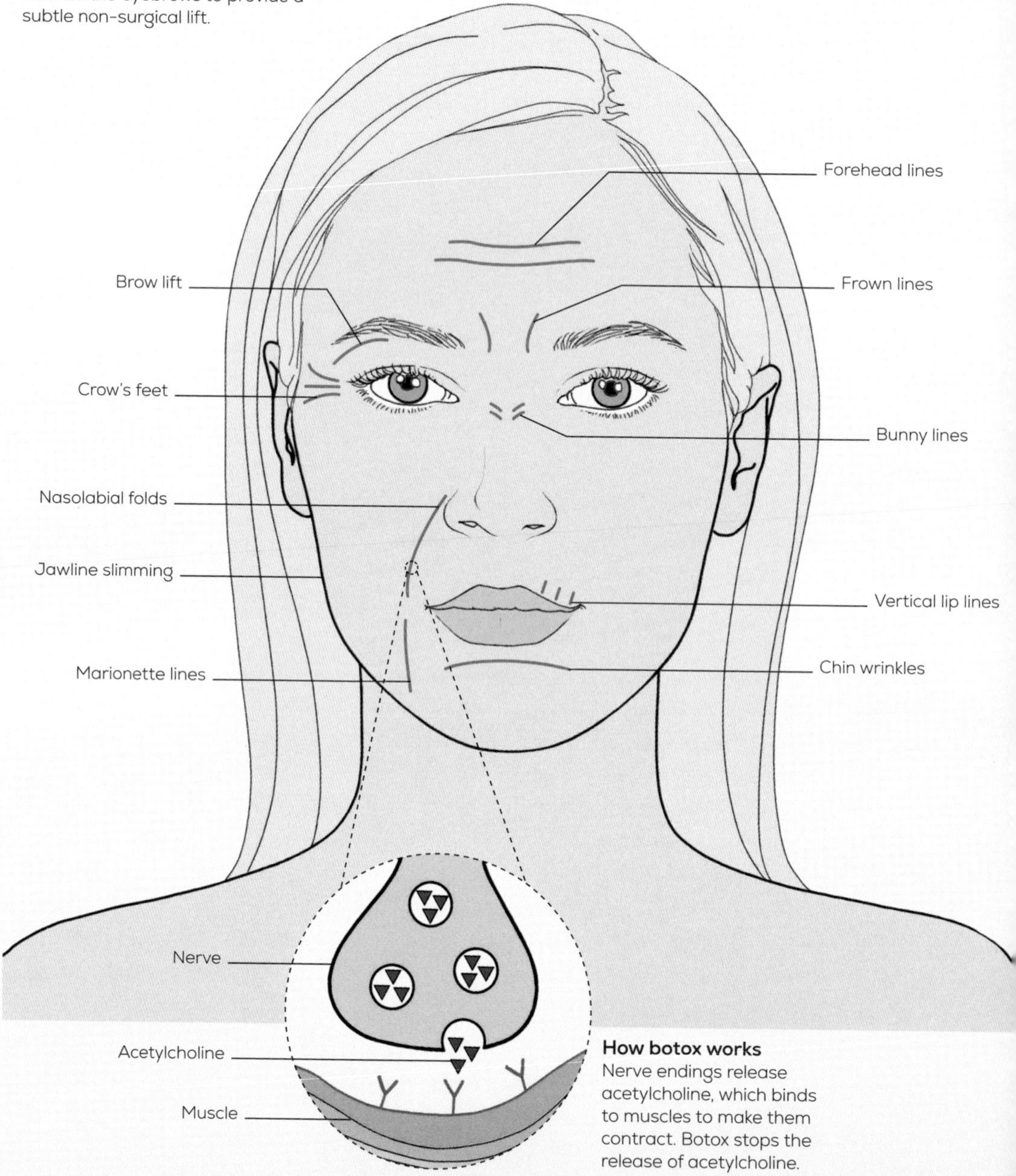

Forehead lines

Brow lift

Frown lines

Crow's feet

Bunny lines

Nasolabial folds

Jawline slimming

Vertical lip lines

Marionette lines

Chin wrinkles

Nerve

Acetylcholine

Muscle

How botox works

Nerve endings release acetylcholine, which binds to muscles to make them contract. Botox stops the release of acetylcholine.

What does botox do?

Botulinum toxin (commonly referred to as botox) is the most toxic substance known to science – and millions of us inject it into our faces every year.

It's a mixture of proteins produced by bacteria like *Clostridium botulinum*, which causes botulism in poorly preserved canned food.

Botox blocks nerves from releasing the neurotransmitters that cause muscle contraction, paralyzing the muscle. It was originally used to treat overactive muscles and spasms. In the early 1990s, some ophthalmologists noticed that patients treated for eyelid spasms also had fewer frown lines. This inspired the development of anti-wrinkle injections, which are now the most common cosmetic procedure worldwide.

As a cosmetic treatment, botox is mostly used to soften dynamic wrinkles that appear when muscles contract, like frown lines and crow's feet. While botox won't work on static wrinkles that are visible when your muscles are relaxed, it can slow down how quickly they become etched into skin. It can also be used to reduce excessive sweating, gummy smiles, and large masseter muscles.

The amount of botox required depends on the strength of the muscle being treated. The paralytic effect reaches a maximum about two weeks after injection, and will last around 3–5 months until the nerve recovers and can activate the muscle again.

Cosmetic botox treatments use very small doses, so they are generally safe and not very painful. The main side effect is paralysis of other muscles if the botox migrates, which can lead to eyelid drooping, downturned lips, or asymmetry, which usually wears off after a couple of weeks. Other possible side effects include temporary bruising, swelling, and botox resistance – where increasingly large doses are needed. It's a cliché that botox will freeze your face and stop you from making facial expressions – practitioners can inject carefully to ensure a natural effect.

BEAUTY MYTHS

PREVENTATIVE BOTOX

"Preventative botox" has been increasingly marketed on social media, which raises questions about our society's relationship with aging, realistic expectations of our appearance, and exploitation of insecurities for profit. While reducing facial movement can theoretically reduce future wrinkles, botox's effects are temporary, so it's likely an unnecessary investment of money when you're younger.

Can skincare products harm my skin?

It's extremely unlikely that skincare products will cause long-term damage to your skin, provided you follow the instructions and the products are made following standard practices.

However, there are some situations where skincare products can temporarily cause negative effects like irritation.

Overuse

When testing for skin tolerance, it's common for companies to test the one product alone, rather than in a skincare routine with multiple products. If three products recommended for "nightly use" are used together, it may cause irritation. Complex skincare routines with multiple active ingredients that all thin the stratum corneum are a common issue. Overuse of these products can impair the ability of your skin to act as a barrier, leading to easily irritated skin that might sting or turn red with products it normally tolerates, or even just water. Your skin might become dry, rough, tight, and uncomfortable. This is sometimes referred to as "sensitized skin", and recovery can take at least two weeks as the stratum corneum needs to be replaced (see pp54–55).

Sun sensitivity

Some ingredients like glycolic and lactic acid are also known to increase sun

HOW TO REDUCE IRRITATION

Ingredients that commonly cause irritation include retinoids, vitamin C, exfoliants, and hydroquinone. Follow these steps to reduce the chances of skin irritation when using new products.

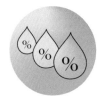

Start with a lower concentration and build up.

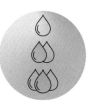

Start applying at a lower frequency e.g. once a week, before building up.

Start with a lower amount and build up.

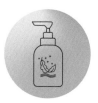

Use non-irritating products in the rest of your routine e.g. gentle cleanser and rich moisturizer.

sensitivity. There is usually a warning on the label to use along with sun protection. The sun sensitivity can persist for over a week after you stop using them.

Can skincare products cause pimples?

Skincare products can contribute to clogged pores and pimples. However, the way an ingredient interacts with an individual's skin oils and follicles is highly personal, and is influenced strongly by the overall formulation. That's why comedogenicity ingredient ratings can't predict which products to use or avoid. If you notice certain products causing a breakout, it can be useful to keep track of ingredients that might be contributing.

Poorly preserved products

Some products may have an ineffective preservative system or may have been improperly stored, so they can decompose or become contaminated with microbes before their expiry date. Using these can lead to rashes and infections. Don't use a product that has changed drastically in colour, texture, or smell, or if there are any visible growths.

BEAUTY MYTHS

RUNNING OUT OF SKIN CELLS

Each time normal cells divide, their DNA shortens slightly. It's believed that once the DNA shortens too much (past the telomeres), the cells become abnormal, which contributes to aging. Since some skin-renewing ingredients increase epidermal turnover, there has been speculation that skin cells may divide too quickly and speed up DNA shortening, so you "run out of skin cells" at a younger age. However, this is a myth. The epidermis is produced by stem cells, which do not experience DNA shortening with division, so this is not a big concern.

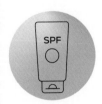

Use adequate sun protection to reduce inflammation from UV.

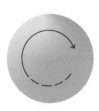

Look for a formula with a gentler delivery system e.g. slow release.

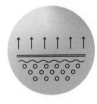

Wait for skin to dry before application to reduce additional penetration with hydration.

Use ingredients that can reduce irritation e.g. antioxidants, panthenol, allantoin.

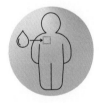

If your skin is sensitive, test new products out on a small area and keep track of products that cause reactions.

Why do wrinkles form?

Wrinkles are an inevitable part of growing older, as internal and external influences change the structure of our skin.

Changes in the dermis in combination with repeated movement are the main cause of deep wrinkles. Collagen, which gives the skin much of its strength, decreases from about age 30. Sun exposure also increases the activity of enzymes which decompose collagen and elastin.

The structure of the dermis also becomes more disorganized as collagen and elastin fibres collect irregularities over time. These occur due to free radicals from metabolic processes and environmental stresses, and attachment of sugars (glycation). UV also creates abnormal masses of elastin, which leads to deep wrinkling (solar elastosis). Together, these lead to a thinner, more uneven dermis that doesn't support the upper layers as effectively, manifesting in wrinkles and lines on the surface. These dermal changes also make the skin less resilient to repeated creasing, which etches wrinkles into the skin over time.

Barrier cells are continuously produced and sloughed off in the epidermis, but this skin turnover process slows and becomes less uniform as we age. Skin also becomes less capable of retaining water. These changes also make the surface of the skin rougher, so wrinkles look more pronounced (see also pp64–65).

Additionally, decreased fat, muscle, and bone in the face causes skin to be stretched less tightly.

Skin over the decades
This graph highlights the profound transformations our skin undergoes with time, charting variations in skin's properties and components.

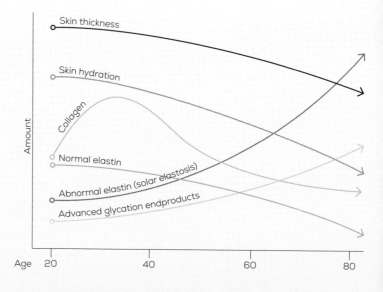

Amount

Skin thickness

Skin hydration

Collagen

Normal elastin

Abnormal elastin (solar elastosis)

Advanced glycation endproducts

Age   20   40   60   80

Collagen, which gives
the skin much of its
strength, decreases
from about age 30.

How do I prevent wrinkles?

Wrinkles are one of the most common reasons for using skincare products. While inevitable, there are many proven ways to reduce their appearance.

We increasingly see celebrities looking baby-faced well into their 50s and 60s, which can make us more self-conscious about our own wrinkles and look for solutions. Remember that celebrities spend huge amounts of money on surgeries and high-end treatments to look that way. It is impossible to fully eradicate wrinkles, but these tips can reduce their appearance, or prevent further wrinkles forming.

Sun protection

The main preventable cause of premature wrinkling is sun exposure. Sunscreen and other forms of sun protection are recommended when going outdoors. There can also be substantial UV exposure in sunny spots indoors, since UVA can pass through glass. Several cases of severe wrinkling on one side of the face have been reported due to indoor sun exposure, particularly inside cars. Avoiding other environmental sources of oxidative stress like smoking and pollution is also beneficial.

Skincare

Moisturizers help the upper layers of skin retain water, which plumps up the skin and makes fine lines and wrinkles shallower. A few active ingredients (see left) have been

Retinoids
Some retinoids like tretinoin, tazarotene, and retinol can increase collagen production, prevent breakdown of dermal proteins, and increase skin turnover.

Hydroxy acids
Chemical exfoliants can smooth out superficial skin layers. At higher concentrations in chemical peels, they can also stimulate collagen and improve elastin quality.

Antioxidants
Some antioxidants may prevent or reverse skin changes linked to oxidative stress. The evidence is strongest for ascorbic acid (vitamin C), which can increase collagen and reduce wrinkles.

Other ingredients
There is some promising data on niacinamide and peptides reducing wrinkles.

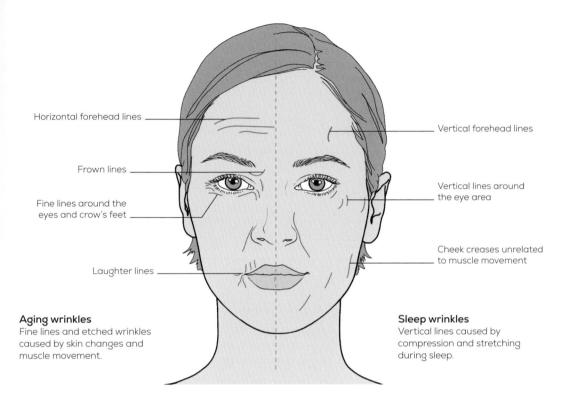

Horizontal forehead lines

Vertical forehead lines

Frown lines

Vertical lines around the eye area

Fine lines around the eyes and crow's feet

Laughter lines

Cheek creases unrelated to muscle movement

Aging wrinkles
Fine lines and etched wrinkles caused by skin changes and muscle movement.

Sleep wrinkles
Vertical lines caused by compression and stretching during sleep.

shown to thicken the dermis and reduce sun damage. Many of these also have effects on the epidermis, which helps reduce wrinkles too.

Skincare products take a while to impact the dermis, so visible changes may take 6–12 months of consistent use.

Clinical treatments

Clinical treatments (see also pp102–103) can stimulate dermal growth and repair processes, often by causing controlled damage to trigger the skin's healing response. This includes chemical peels, microneedling, light treatments (lasers, LED, IPL), and "skin tightening" radiofrequency and ultrasound treatments.

Fillers can be injected to fill in wrinkles and stimulate the synthesis of dermal collagen. Botox can reduce muscle movements and stop dynamic wrinkles from becoming visible when the muscles aren't active.

Other changes

Vertical lines called sleep wrinkles can form from pressing your face into a pillow when you sleep. These can be reduced by sleeping in a position that puts less pressure on the face, such as on your back.

There's some evidence that a healthy lifestyle, with a balanced, nutritious diet, regular exercise, adequate sleep, and less stress can reduce inflammation and slow down age-related skin changes.

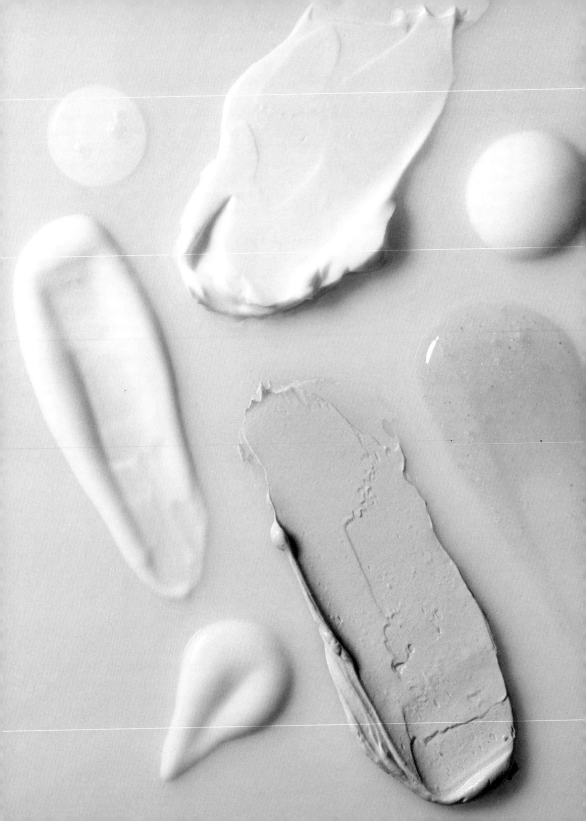

Moisturizers help
the upper layers of
skin retain water, which
plumps up the skin and
makes fine lines and
wrinkles shallower.

Can I reduce cellulite?

Cellulite refers to textured or dimpled skin, commonly around the thighs and buttocks.

Cellulite is caused by increased subcutaneous fat, a weakened dermis, and thicker fibrous bands (septae) under the skin. Genetics, hormones, poor circulation, fluid retention, and inflammation can all contribute. These factors are far more common in women – an estimated 80 to 95% of women have some cellulite.

While cellulite is normal female physiology, some people want to reduce its appearance. Many "anti-cellulite" creams make overblown claims. These can have a temporary effect because they are applied via massage, which increases circulation and mobilizes retained fluid. In other words, it is the massage that helps the skin's appearance, rather than the cream itself. Caffeine and theobromine creams could potentially reduce fat but are unlikely to penetrate deep enough. Retinoids can help modestly by strengthening the dermis.

Long-term results can only be achieved by clinical interventions. Cutting the underlying septae (subcision) allows fat to spread out more evenly, giving dramatic and long-lasting results. Liposuction (fat removal) and treatments like radiofrequency or laser can also reduce cellulite permanently.

Formation of cellulite
In cellulite, increased subcutaneous fat bulges out through a weakened dermis to create an uneven surface. Fibrous, thickened septae pull skin inwards to cause deep indented dimples.

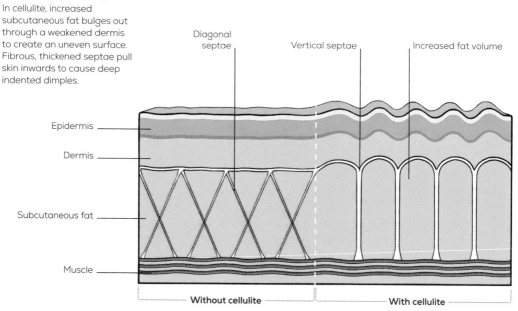

Diagonal septae

Vertical septae

Increased fat volume

Epidermis

Dermis

Subcutaneous fat

Muscle

Without cellulite

With cellulite

How can I treat dark spots and uneven pigment?

Uneven pigment is a very common occurrence in non-white skin, especially with advancing age. The most common issue is hyperpigmentation, where areas of skin have excessive pigment.

Hyperpigmentation includes:
- Melasma: large, irregular patches of pigment particularly on the cheeks.
- Post-inflammatory hyperpigmentation (PIH) that forms after trauma, like wounds or acne.
- Solar lentigines (sun spots).
- Periorbital pigmentation around the eyes.

How does pigmentation form?

Melanin pigment is produced in the melanocyte cells at the base of the epidermis. Melanocytes contain small structures called melanosomes. Inside them, the amino acid tyrosine is converted to melanin, then the pigmented melanosomes are transferred to keratinocytes, which gradually rise to the surface. Disrupting the bottom of the epidermis can cause melanin to deposit in the deeper dermis, which is more difficult to remove. Shallower pigment tends to look more brown, while dermal pigment looks blue or grey.

Oestrogen can also cause hyperpigmentation, and melasma during pregnancy. Oral contraceptives have also been known to cause pigmentation. Treating irregular pigmentation usually involves both preventing the formation of excess pigment, and removing existing pigment. Some forms of pigmentation can be very stubborn, so multiple forms of treatment are often combined.

Prevention

Pigment is removed as keratinocytes shed, so preventing excess pigment production can be enough to fade hyperpigmentation. However, deeper pigmentation may not shed as easily, or as quickly. It typically takes at least eight weeks for preventative pigment treatments to cause visible changes.

Most pigment treatments will not affect normal pigment production, but illegal bleaching creams with ingredients like mercury can damage skin. Preventative treatments generally target the following three steps of pigment development.

Reduce melanocyte stimulation

The sun is the main environmental cause of excess pigment formation, so preventing sun exposure and using a high protection sunscreen daily is key to preventing and reducing hyperpigmentation. Tinted products can protect against the intense blue light from the sun, while also disguising pigment.

Inflammation can also trigger hyperpigmentation. Treat any underlying cause of inflammation, such as acne (see pp118–119), and use gentle skincare products with barrier-protecting ingredients. Antioxidants (see p28) can reduce both inflammation and sun-induced pigment. Ironically, many pigment treatments irritate the skin and can cause inflammation, which can lead to rebound pigmentation. Glucocorticosteroids are sometimes prescribed to reduce inflammation.

> Ironically, many pigment treatments irritate the skin and can cause inflammation, which can lead to rebound pigmentation.

Reduce melanin production

The main enzyme involved in melanin production is tyrosinase, so ingredients that prevent it from working (tyrosinase inhibitors) are some of the most successful pigment treatments.

Hydroquinone is the "gold standard" treatment for hyperpigmentation and is a very effective tyrosinase inhibitor. It can also kill melanocyte cells and destroy melanosomes. Side effects like irritation, lighter patches, and dark pigmentation (ochronosis) are more common at higher concentrations and with prolonged continuous use, so a one-month break

is often recommended every three months. Other ingredients popular in skincare that interfere with melanin production include cysteamine, azelaic acid, kojic acid, ascorbic acid, arbutin, and glabridin.

Reduce transfer to keratinocytes

Blocking the transfer of melanosomes to keratinocytes can reduce pigmentation. Niacinamide and soy extracts are thought to work in this way.

Speed up pigment removal

Increasing the rate of skin turnover speeds up the shedding of epidermal pigment. This is how retinoids and exfoliants like glycolic acid and salicylic acid work. They can also help to prevent acne, a common cause of PIH.

Peels can quickly remove pigment in the top layers of skin, but the risk of rebound pigmentation is high if not performed carefully.

Triple combination creams contain a retinoid, a corticosteroid, and a tyrosinase inhibitor. They work synergistically to target different parts of the pigmentation cycle and offset each other's side effects. A common combination is 0.05% tretinoin, 0.01% fluocinolone acetonide, and 4% hydroquinone.

Laser treatments (see pp125–127) are commonly used to break up melanin pigment in both the epidermis and dermis, and can induce skin cells to shed faster. As laser treatments can cause inflammation, rebound hyperpigmentation is a possible side effect. Gentler laser technologies like picosecond and Nd:YAG lasers are lower risk, and tyrosinase inhibitors can be used preventatively before treatment.

HOW PIGMENT FORMS

Treatments that even out excess pigment target one or more steps in the melanin production process.

1 Melanocytes are stimulated

Melanin-producing cells at the base of the epidermis are triggered, such as by hormones, inflammation, or UV.

2 Melanin pigment is produced inside melanosomes

Colourless precursors are transformed into melanin pigment by enzymes including tyrosinase. This occurs inside packets called melanosomes.

3 Melanosomes are transferred to keratinocyte cells

The pigmented melanosomes are distributed into keratinocyte skin cells to produce skin colour.

4 Melanin is removed when dead skin cells are shed

Keratinocytes move upwards through the epidermis, and shed along with the pigment they contain when they reach the surface.

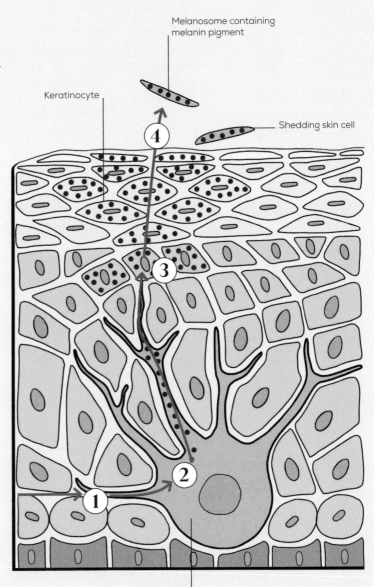

Melanosome containing melanin pigment

Keratinocyte

Shedding skin cell

Melanocyte

How do I deal with pimples and acne?

Acne is an extremely common skin condition that affects around 80% of people at some point, and it's one of the main reasons people use skincare products.

Why do pimples form?

There are four major contributors to acne: high sebum production, increased pore clogging (due to differences in sebum composition and shedding of dead skin cells), overgrowth of *Cutibacterium acnes* bacteria, and inflammation. These can all be influenced by genetics, as well as hormonal medications like anabolic steroids and contraceptives, and conditions like polycystic ovarian syndrome (PCOS). Skincare and lifestyle habits can also contribute, as they can cause clogged pores and inflammation.

A pimple starts when a hair follicle's opening (pore) becomes clogged with a microscopic plug of dead skin cells and hardened sebum (microcomedone). As it gets larger, it becomes a whitehead if it stays under the skin, or a blackhead if it is exposed to oxygen and darkens.

Sebum can then build up behind the clog, swelling the follicle. Acne bacteria feed off sebum and multiply, leading to inflammation, redness, and pus. This can build up and rupture into the surrounding skin, causing scars. Acne tends to start in adolescence when sebum production surges. However, adult acne is also common, especially in women.

Treatments for acne

Acne treatments target one or more of the four main contributors to acne. It is usually better to use them continuously to prevent microcomedones from forming.

Acne can be a stubborn, recurring condition. You may need to try several treatments before seeing results, or use them in tandem. If you aren't seeing improvement after trying several options, or your acne is causing distress or scarring, it's a good idea to seek medical advice.

Retinoids treat acne by normalizing skin turnover. Drug retinoids tretinoin and adapalene are more effective than cosmetic retinoids like retinaldehyde and retinol. Isotretinoin is an oral medication that also reduces sebum production.

Over-the-counter benzoyl peroxide products kill acne bacteria and reduce clogged pores. Studies have found that leave-on products with 2.5% work as well as 10%, but with less irritation. Benzoyl peroxide can bleach fabrics, but this can be reduced by using it in wash-off products. However, benzoyl peroxide can inactivate some ingredients, including many retinoids.

Chemical exfoliants help skin cells slough off and can reduce pore clogging. Salicylic acid is particularly well-studied in acne and has anti-inflammatory effects as well. Azelaic acid is a gentle option with

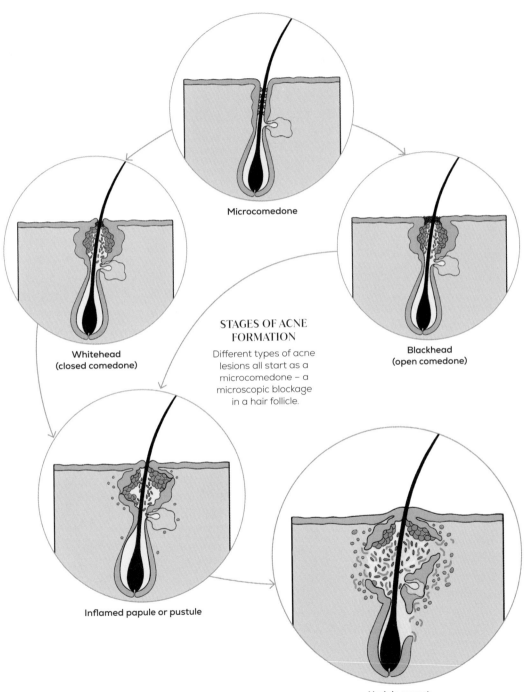

Microcomedone

Whitehead
(closed comedone)

Blackhead
(open comedone)

STAGES OF ACNE FORMATION

Different types of acne lesions all start as a microcomedone – a microscopic blockage in a hair follicle.

Inflamed papule or pustule

Nodule or cyst

antimicrobial, exfoliating and anti-inflammatory properties, but typically takes longer to work. Sulfur is also antibacterial.

Oral or topical antibiotics can be prescribed to reduce acne bacteria, but are usually combined with another treatment to avoid antimicrobial resistance.

Prescription hormonal treatments can address underlying hormonal factors and reduce sebum production. These can be oral medications (contraceptives containing oestrogen and anti-androgenic progestins, spironolactone) or topical creams (clascoterone).

Microneedle pimple patches deliver anti-acne ingredients deeper into skin. Hydrocolloid bandages can protect open pimples from infection, speed up healing, and block UV.

The relationship between diet and acne is complex (see pp74–75). While some people may benefit from dietary changes, it's generally more reliable to use other treatments.

Clinical treatments that have shown success for acne include chemical peels and blue light. Corticosteroids can be injected to flatten cysts quickly. Studies have found modest benefits with home light devices, but these are relatively expensive.

ROUTINE FOR ACNE PRONE SKIN

Harsh skincare products can exacerbate acne. A preventative routine for acne-prone skin should include the following.

Gentle cleansing
Use a gentle low-pH cleanser to remove sebum, dead cells, and dirt without disrupting skin.

Applying sunscreen
UV can kill bacteria and temporarily reduce pimples, but usually worsens acne by causing inflammation. It also darkens post-inflammatory hyperpigmentation.

Moisturizing
Since acne treatments are often irritating, it's important to adequately moisturize your skin.

Exfoliating once a week
Reduce clogged pores by using an exfoliant like salicylic acid regularly.

Should I pop my pimples?

Popping can rupture pimples, spreading the infection deeper into the skin and causing more severe scarring. It's best not to pop pimples, but if necessary:
- Clean the area and your hands.
- Only squeeze pimples with visible pus.
- Lance the pimple with a sterile needle at an angle (to avoid introducing the infection deeper).
- Squeeze with very gentle pressure.
- Stop squeezing when all the pus is out, or when clear liquid or blood emerges.
- Clean and protect the wound with a bandage such as a hydrocolloid.

How do I fade scars?

Scars occur when deeper skin layers are injured, and there is a visible difference between the new tissue and the surrounding skin.

They are often caused by acne, injury, or surgery. Scars can be raised or depressed, and are often coloured.

Reducing scars during healing

Scarring depends largely on genetics, but certain practices can support healing and make scars less noticeable.

- Keep the injury clean and moist.
- Stretching the skin can enlarge a wound and cause a bigger scar. Stitches should not be removed prematurely.
- Topical products can interfere with healing – don't use them until skin is healed over.
- Protect the wound from the sun with a bandage.

Fading scars

Silicone gel or sheets can help flatten raised scars. In darker skin, wounds can stimulate hyperpigmentation. Pigment-reducing ingredients like hydroquinone and retinoids can be used for a few weeks before surgery. They can be resumed after healing to fade pigment, along with sunscreen and treatments like lasers and peels.

Since scarring usually involves the deeper layers of skin, professional treatments are often required to make scars less visible. Laser resurfacing, chemical peels, dermabrasion, and microneedling are effective for smoothing out widespread shallow scarring, common with acne. Raised scars can be treated with steroids, lasers, or surgery.

Indented scars can be filled with dermal fillers or fat grafts. Smaller deep scars can be treated with trichloroacetic acid. Subcision cuts any scar tissue pulling skin inwards.

TYPES OF SCAR

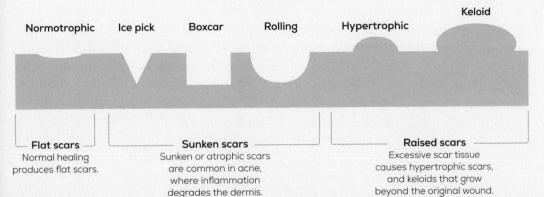

Normotrophic   Ice pick   Boxcar   Rolling   Hypertrophic   Keloid

Flat scars
Normal healing produces flat scars.

Sunken scars
Sunken or atrophic scars are common in acne, where inflammation degrades the dermis.

Raised scars
Excessive scar tissue causes hypertrophic scars, and keloids that grow beyond the original wound.

How can I reduce pores and oil?

Photo manipulation has distorted our expectations of what actual skin looks like. Your pores are much less visible than you think – most people aren't looking as closely as you!

Visible pores are tiny openings in the skin's surface that lead to hair follicles and sebaceous glands. They release oily sebum to keep the skin moisturized.

Causes of enlarged pores and oily skin

Oily skin and enlarged pores are closely linked. The main determinants of oil production and pore size are genetics and hormones, particularly dihydrotestosterone, testosterone, and progesterone. Skin tends to be oilier in warm and humid weather.

Pores usually enlarge with age as the collagen and elastin networks around pores weaken (see pp64–65). Sun damage and other environmental stressors also contribute.

Dead skin cells and oil can clog pores and stretch them out. These plugs darken with exposure to oxygen, which also makes pores more visible.

Treatments

Many anti-acne medications (isotretinoin, spironolactone, oral contraceptives) partly work by reducing oil, which will also reduce pore size. Botox injections and some laser treatments can also decrease oil and pores.

A few skincare ingredients like niacinamide and saw palmetto can potentially reduce oil, but their effects tend to be mild and inconsistent.

Ingredients that keep pores unclogged, like retinoids and chemical exfoliants, can make pores less noticeable. These can also tighten pores by increasing collagen and elastin.

Can steaming clear pores?

Steam is often recommended to "open up pores", but pores don't open and close with heat. Gentle steam can lubricate pores and

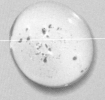

Gentle cleansers
Many people use harsh, irritating cleansers to dry out oily skin. These dehydrate skin, making it feel dry and oily at the same time. Instead, use a gentle cleanser once or twice a day.

Moisturizing humectants
Use moisturizing toners and serums with more humectants and less oils to hydrate skin and reduce tightness and irritation. They also plump up skin around the pores, making them less noticeable.

Remove excess oil
Remove excess oil with translucent powder, clay masks, and blotting papers.

soften sebum, making it easier to extract clogs, but massaging oils into your skin can have a similar effect. Excessive heat can irritate and inflame skin, which enlarges pores in the long run.

Skincare for oily skin
While skincare won't drastically reduce oil production, appropriate products can make oily skin easier to manage (see right). It's a myth that you can "trick" oily skin into producing less sebum with facial oils – there is no mechanism in the skin that will compensate for the amount of surface oil.

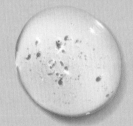

It's a myth that you can "trick" oily skin into producing less sebum with facial oils – there is no mechanism in the skin that will compensate for the amount of surface oil.

How do I treat stretch marks?

Stretch marks (striae) form when rapid growth stretches the skin, causing permanent changes that resemble scar tissue.

Some people are more susceptible to stretch marks, due to hormones or genetics. While stretch marks are a perfectly natural development that affects many people, some people can feel self-conscious about them.

What treatments work?

Treatments can hide stretch marks by thickening the skin (e.g. by increasing collagen), decreasing redness, or changing the pigmentation to match the surrounding skin. A combination of treatments is usually more successful.

- Tretinoin creams increase collagen, but caution is needed during pregnancy.
- Glycolic acid peels can also increase collagen and thicken the epidermis.
- Laser treatments can remove blood vessels in red stretch marks, and increase collagen.
- Radiofrequency and microneedling treatments are becoming more popular, but the evidence is not strong yet.
- Some studies suggest that massage and moisturizers can prevent stretch marks by reducing tension. A few actives like *Centella asiatica* extract and hyaluronic acid can also potentially help.

HOW STRETCH MARKS FORM

Stretch marks commonly form during pregnancy and puberty, as well as with bodybuilding, rapid weight gain, and corticosteroid use. They often develop on the thighs, abdomen, upper arms, breasts, and buttocks.

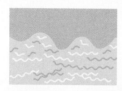

Before tension
Collagen and elastin fibres in the dermis are usually randomly arranged and regular.

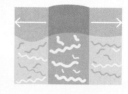

Inflammatory phase
With prolonged tension, skin becomes inflamed and itchy. Collagen and elastin fibres start to break down and reorganize. Stretch marks begin pale, then darken to red. They are often raised due to swelling.

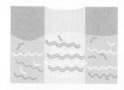

After healing
When no longer under tension, inflammation subsides. Stretch marks become sunken and turn white in pale skin or brown in darker skin, resembling scars.

What do laser and light treatments do?

Light treatments are extremely versatile, and can work under the skin's surface to give rapid results.

Lasers are machines that produce high energy, focused beams of light of specific wavelengths. They are used in many targeted treatments that go beyond the skin's surface and give rapid results, but they can also cause side effects.

How do lasers work?

Different substances in skin (chromophores) absorb different wavelengths of light. The absorbed light turns into a large amount of heat, which can selectively destroy parts of the skin in a process known as selective photothermolysis.

Since lasers operate at specific wavelengths, a specific part of the skin can be targeted with minimal damage to the rest of the skin. The light duration, laser beam pattern, and intensity can also be adjusted to improve targeting.

What can lasers do?

Laser skin treatments commonly target melanin, haemoglobin, or water using different wavelengths. Longer wavelengths can be used to penetrate deeper into skin.

Melanin is targeted to remove unwanted patches of pigment in the epidermis or dermis. Laser hair removal also heats up melanin to kill cells in the hair root. Multiple treatments are required to target hairs in different stages of the growth cycle.

Vascular lasers target haemoglobin in blood to treat telangiectasias (spider veins), port wine stains, angiomas, and rosacea.

Since skin has high water content, laser treatments that target water cause controlled damage to stimulate the skin's renewal processes. This can be used to induce collagen production (laser rejuvenation), or smooth out fine lines and scars (laser resurfacing). Ablative treatments remove the epidermis entirely, which can achieve more dramatic changes but require a longer recovery time (usually over a week), tend to be more painful, and have a higher risk of side effects. Non-ablative lasers leave the surface of the skin intact – for example, they might use a fractionating head to split the beam into smaller spots.

Lasers are also used for tattoo removal. While older methods worked by damaging skin generally, newer techniques are more selective and cause less scarring. However, complete tattoo removal is often not possible.

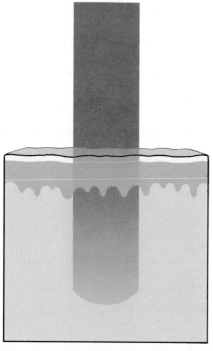

Laser
Lasers deliver high energy,
aligned beams of light with
specific wavelengths.

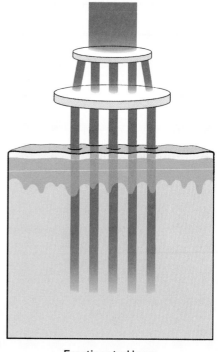

Fractionated laser
A fractionating head splits up the
laser beam, so only a fraction of
the skin is treated.

TYPES OF LIGHT TREATMENTS

Different instruments are used
to impact the skin with various
wavelengths and intensities of light.

Other light treatments

Like lasers, intense pulsed light (IPL)
treatments also work via selective
photothermolysis. However, they use a
broader range of wavelengths that are less
aligned, so they are less targeted and precise
than lasers. They are most commonly used
for removing facial telangiectasias, hair,
and liver spots. LED (light emitting diode)
treatments shine particular light
wavelengths on skin using panels of LED
bulbs. Skin is exposed to light continuously
for around 5–30 minutes, at a lower
intensity than with lasers or IPL.

LED devices can be used for
photodynamic therapy, where light is used
to activate a chemical in the skin. For
example, 5-aminolevulinic acid is applied
to skin, then activated with red light in skin
cancer treatments. Blue light is also used
to treat acne by activating porphyrin
molecules within acne bacteria to
kill them. There are also LED treatments
that work via photobiomodulation, where

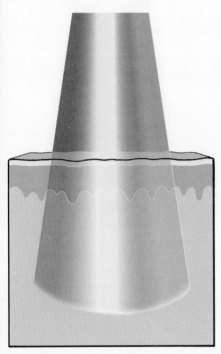

IPL

IPL delivers a broader range of
wavelengths, in short bursts.

RISKS OF LASER AND
LIGHT TREATMENTS

Like with other clinical treatments, light
treatments carry risks and results are often
dependent on the practitioner.

- Check your practitioner's qualifications
  and reviews.

- High intensity light devices can cause pain,
  redness, burns, scars, and pigment changes.
  They can also damage the eyes, so eye
  protection should be worn. In some situations
  the risks of light treatments can be higher, such
  as after taking certain medications or with
  tanned skin.

- Laser and IPL treatments work better with
  more contrast between the target and the
  surrounding skin, so it can be more difficult to
  treat darker skin, which is also more prone to
  pigment changes. However, newer laser
  techniques and instruments can treat darker
  skin more effectively. For example, picosecond
  lasers produce shorter pulses that limit the
  build-up of heat, and use sound energy along
  with heat. Longer wavelengths (e.g. from
  Nd:YAG lasers) can also be used to reduce
  damage to dark skin. Make sure you choose a
  practitioner who has experience in treating skin
  tones similar to yours.

- While home devices are less powerful, they can
  still cause injury, especially if they are misused,
  or aren't well maintained and become faulty.

the wavelengths cause a change in the
biological functioning of skin cells. The two
most commonly used wavelengths are red
light at 633 nm and near-infrared light at
830 nm, which stimulate the wound-healing
response. LED treatments have been used
successfully to rejuvenate skin and treat a
range of conditions including acne, psoriasis,
and dissecting scalp cellulitis.

UV phototherapy is used to treat some
skin conditions like psoriasis, atopic
dermatitis, and skin cancers. It mostly works
by suppressing inflammation and reducing
immune activity.

The two commonly used LED
wavelengths stimulate the
wound-healing response.

Can I recreate clinical treatments at home?

Many home devices attempt to replicate in-clinic treatments, with varying degrees of success. Check that devices comply with regulations in your region before purchasing.

ELECTRONIC DEVICES

Home electronic devices are typically weaker than in-clinic treatments, but can give benefits with consistent use.

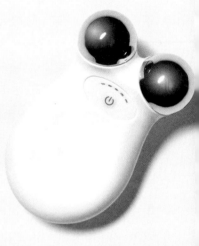

Microcurrent devices

These use a weak electric current to stimulate and firm muscles for a temporarily "lifted" effect. Since they act on muscles, they can work deeper than most skincare products, but the effect is more modest than clinical treatments and requires consistent use to maintain.

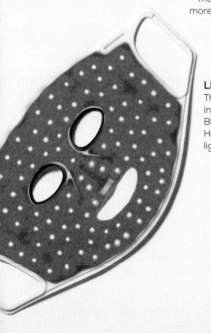

LED devices

These use light (usually red or near-infrared) to stimulate skin healing. Blue light devices are used for acne. Home devices produce less intense light, but eye protection is still advised.

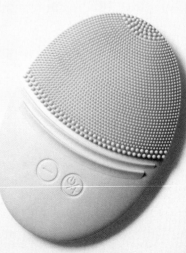

Vibrating or rotating brushes

Used to clean and exfoliate, but they are irritating if used too frequently or with strong pressure. Silicone brushes are usually easier to clean. Some brushes claim to stimulate collagen or push actives into skin, but there is little evidence for these benefits.

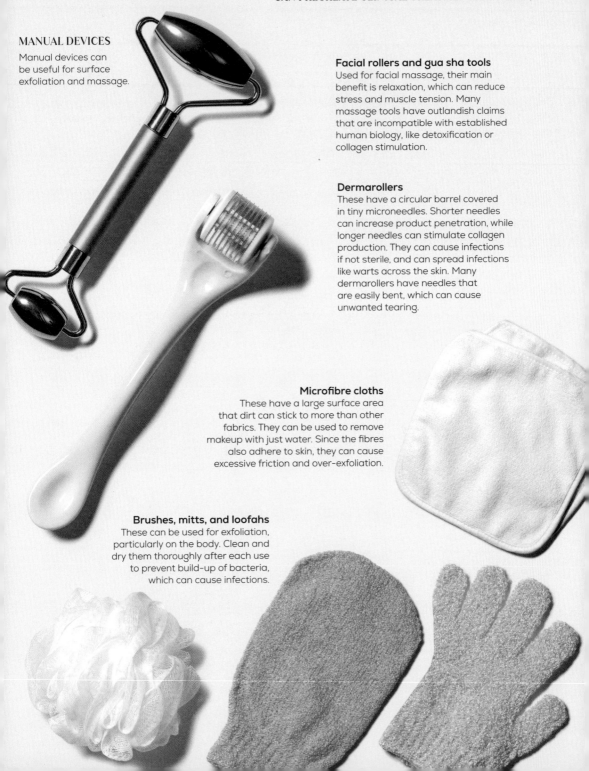

MANUAL DEVICES

Manual devices can
be useful for surface
exfoliation and massage.

Facial rollers and gua sha tools

Used for facial massage, their main
benefit is relaxation, which can reduce
stress and muscle tension. Many
massage tools have outlandish claims
that are incompatible with established
human biology, like detoxification or
collagen stimulation.

Dermarollers

These have a circular barrel covered
in tiny microneedles. Shorter needles
can increase product penetration, while
longer needles can stimulate collagen
production. They can cause infections
if not sterile, and can spread infections
like warts across the skin. Many
dermarollers have needles that
are easily bent, which can cause
unwanted tearing.

Microfibre cloths

These have a large surface area
that dirt can stick to more than other
fabrics. They can be used to remove
makeup with just water. Since the fibres
also adhere to skin, they can cause
excessive friction and over-exfoliation.

Brushes, mitts, and loofahs

These can be used for exfoliation,
particularly on the body. Clean and
dry them thoroughly after each use
to prevent build-up of bacteria,
which can cause infections.

How do artificial tanning products work?

Fake tan products come in many forms, like lotions, foams, and sprays, but they all contain the key ingredients dihydroxyacetone and erythrulose. These react with proteins in the stratum corneum to produce brown compounds called melanoidins. The reaction is similar to browning of bread via the Maillard reaction.

Dihydroxyacetone is more common in fake tans. It reacts with skin to give a slightly orange tan within eight hours, with the full tan developing after about a day. Greenish-brown dyes are often added to artificial tanning products to create a more natural tone.

Erythrulose reacts more slowly with skin, giving a more natural-looking but lighter tan colour that develops after 24 hours.

Fake tans fade as the stained dead skin cells slough off, and typically last 5–7 days. Gradual tanners contain lower active concentrations, so regular use maintains a longer-lasting tanned look.

Fake tan timeline
The colour of your fake tan comes from the combined action of these ingredients. Dyes give a green-toned guide colour that comes off after washing. Dihydroxyacetone reacts to form an orange-toned tan, while erythrulose creates a more natural, longer-lasting brown colour.

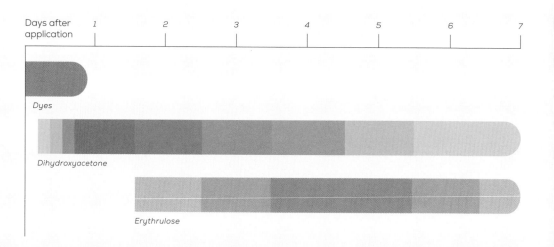

Days after application	1	2	3	4	5	6	7

Dyes

Dihydroxyacetone

Erythrulose

BEAUTY MYTHS

TANNING DRUGS

Some injectable and inhalable "tanning drugs" can stimulate melanocytes to produce more melanin. These are often sold illegally under names like "Melanotan", and have not been tested for safety. There have been reports of concerning side effects like nausea and flushing, and they are suspected to have contributed to some cases of melanoma.

HOW CAN I GET A MORE EVEN LOOKING FAKE TAN?

Regardless of the type of tanning product you choose, there are some steps you can take before, during, and after application to ensure a flawless finish.

Exfoliate

Fake tan reacts with dead skin, so any build-up can give an uneven finish. Exfoliate your skin thoroughly before tanning, especially your knees, elbows, and ankles.

Moisturize

Moisturize your skin every day after application to help the tan wear off evenly. Many fake tan formulas dry out your skin, leading to disrupted skin turnover.

Use special mitts and tools

These can help you apply the product more smoothly. Mousses and sprays are also easier to spread. Gradual tanners that build up over several applications can help prevent patchiness.

Avoid water

Water exposure can cause fake tans to streak. It's generally advised to wait at least eight hours before showering after a spray tan. However, some formulations are specifically designed to work faster, or can even be used in the shower.

Do skin supplements work?

In general, there's little evidence that dietary supplements are beneficial if you have an adequate diet.

There's some evidence that particular supplements can have additional benefits for skin. However, there aren't many high quality or independent studies available, and the evidence that does exist is often mixed, potentially due to variation in people's diets and in supplement composition. Supplements are not well standardized, and changes in production can have large impacts on their composition and absorption, particularly if they're naturally sourced.

Supplements also carry more risks than food sources. There can be contamination issues, and some ingredients beneficial in food can even be detrimental when taken alone in large quantities. Avoid brands with a history of poor quality in tests from independent labs.

It's also worth noting that it's almost always less efficient to get a substance to your skin by taking it orally, than by applying it topically. Supplements need to be absorbed from the digestive system into blood before being distributed around the body, and your skin is at the very edge. Their effects on skin are generally milder and less universal than topical treatments.

Sun protection

The most promising supplements are for sun protection. Niacinamide (vitamin B3) has been found to reduce new non-melanoma skin cancers in high-risk patients, such as those who have already been treated for cancer or have a family history.

Some antioxidant supplements have reduced sunburn in studies, and could be useful for people with very sun-sensitive skin. These include vitamin C, vitamin E, carotenoids (lycopene, beta-carotene, astaxanthin), plant polyphenols (e.g. from green tea), and a *Polypodium* fern extract. However, their benefits are not well substantiated compared to other sun protective measures, so they should not be considered substitutes for limiting the UV that reaches the skin in the first place (see p84).

Skincare supplements

Here are some common supplements and their potential
benefits – the evidence for their effectiveness is mixed.

SUPPLEMENT		TYPICAL DOSE USED IN STUDIES	POTENTIAL SKIN BENEFITS
Niacinamide		500mg twice daily	Skin cancer protection
Collagen		2.5–5g daily	Skin hydration and elasticity
Polypodium fern extract		240mg twice daily	UV protection
Carotenoids		15–180mg daily	UV protection
Probiotics (some strains)		Variable	Atopic dermatitis, acne, skin hydration
Omega-3 fatty acids (EPA, DHA)		1–4g daily	Dry skin and inflammatory conditions

Antioxidants

Antioxidants have also been studied for improving age-related skin changes like dryness, elasticity, and wrinkles, as well as inflammatory conditions like psoriasis. These studies used the same antioxidants investigated for sun protection, as well as others including curcumin, resveratrol, and zinc.

However, antioxidant supplementation is not without risk. Oxidative stress has many important functions in the body that can potentially be disturbed by antioxidant supplementation. For example, in some studies, antioxidant supplements increased the growth of cancer cells. Fruits and vegetables are a safer way to boost your antioxidant intake.

Collagen

Collagen peptides (hydrolyzed collagen) are produced by breaking down collagen from fish and beef, and have had beneficial effects on skin in clinical trials. They contain hydroxyproline, an amino acid that's relatively unique to collagen. It's thought that collagen peptides are small enough to absorb through the gut and signal to skin to increase hydration and elasticity, and produce more collagen. However, many varieties of collagen peptides on the market

aren't supported by good evidence, and they tend to be poor value for money compared to well-established skincare products.

Probiotics

There is promising research on the influence of microbiome on skin. However, the vast number of species present and their variation from person to person makes it difficult to find suitable treatments.

Studies on various probiotic supplements ("friendly" bacteria) for atopic dermatitis have been mixed, with some finding benefits while others have found little improvement. Some evidence suggests that they could be helpful for acne. Probiotics in creams may be more effective, but investigations are very preliminary.

Fatty acids and oils

Omega-3 essential fatty acids can't be synthesized in the body and must be obtained from the diet. They are needed to produce epidermal lipid matrix components like ceramides, and can also have an anti-inflammatory effect. In some studies, omega-3 supplements have been found to help with dry skin and inflammatory skin conditions such as atopic dermatitis, psoriasis, and acne.

Collagen supplements tend to be poor value for money compared to well-established skincare products.

How do I look after my skin in winter?

Skin tends to dry out more in winter and become itchy, so many people will need to change their skincare routines.

Itchy winter skin

Harsh environmental conditions in winter reduce the skin's water and oil content. Low humidity and wind can make skin lose moisture faster. Heaters can also dry out skin, and hot showers can wash away the skin's natural moisturizers.

This means your skin is less resilient and can't recover as easily from the same sorts of impacts. Its normal functions are disrupted, leading to flaky, cracked skin that's tight, red, and itchy.

Cracked skin on feet

Dead skin often builds up on feet as a protective response to friction. However, this can get too thick, crack, and become painful.

You can remove dead skin with abrasive tools like files or pumice stones. Soak your feet in warm water before removal to soften dead skin and prevent cracking. Be careful not to cut into living layers as this can cause infection. A podiatrist can also shave away dead skin, and remove any corns or calluses.

Exfoliating and moisturizing products can keep dead cells sloughing off and maintain softer feet. Many foot creams contain urea, a humectant moisturizer that also helps break down dead skin. Foot peels containing hydroxy acid exfoliants inside plastic "socks" can be used every few months.

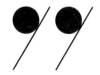

The harsher environmental conditions in winter can mean that your skin is less resilient and can't recover as easily.

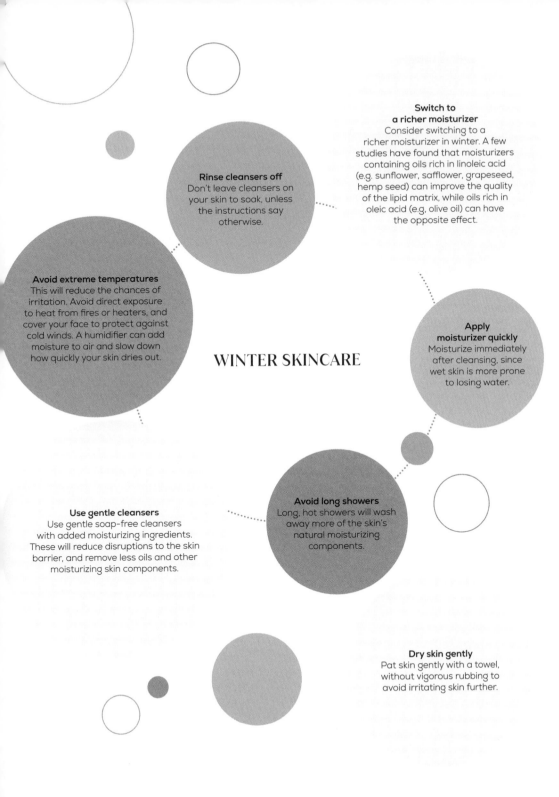

**Switch to
a richer moisturizer**
Consider switching to a
richer moisturizer in winter. A few
studies have found that moisturizers
containing oils rich in linoleic acid
(e.g. sunflower, safflower, grapeseed,
hemp seed) can improve the quality
of the lipid matrix, while oils rich in
oleic acid (e.g. olive oil) can have
the opposite effect.

Rinse cleansers off
Don't leave cleansers on
your skin to soak, unless
the instructions say
otherwise.

Avoid extreme temperatures
This will reduce the chances of
irritation. Avoid direct exposure
to heat from fires or heaters, and
cover your face to protect against
cold winds. A humidifier can add
moisture to air and slow down
how quickly your skin dries out.

WINTER SKINCARE

**Apply
moisturizer quickly**
Moisturize immediately
after cleansing, since
wet skin is more prone
to losing water.

Use gentle cleansers
Use gentle soap-free cleansers
with added moisturizing ingredients.
These will reduce disruptions to the skin
barrier, and remove less oils and other
moisturizing skin components.

Avoid long showers
Long, hot showers will wash
away more of the skin's
natural moisturizing
components.

Dry skin gently
Pat skin gently with a towel,
without vigorous rubbing to
avoid irritating skin further.

Hair

Structure of hair

Our hair's structure explains how it behaves, and how best to look after it. Each hair has a protective cuticle wrapped around a cortex, containing bundles of keratin surrounded by keratin-associated proteins.

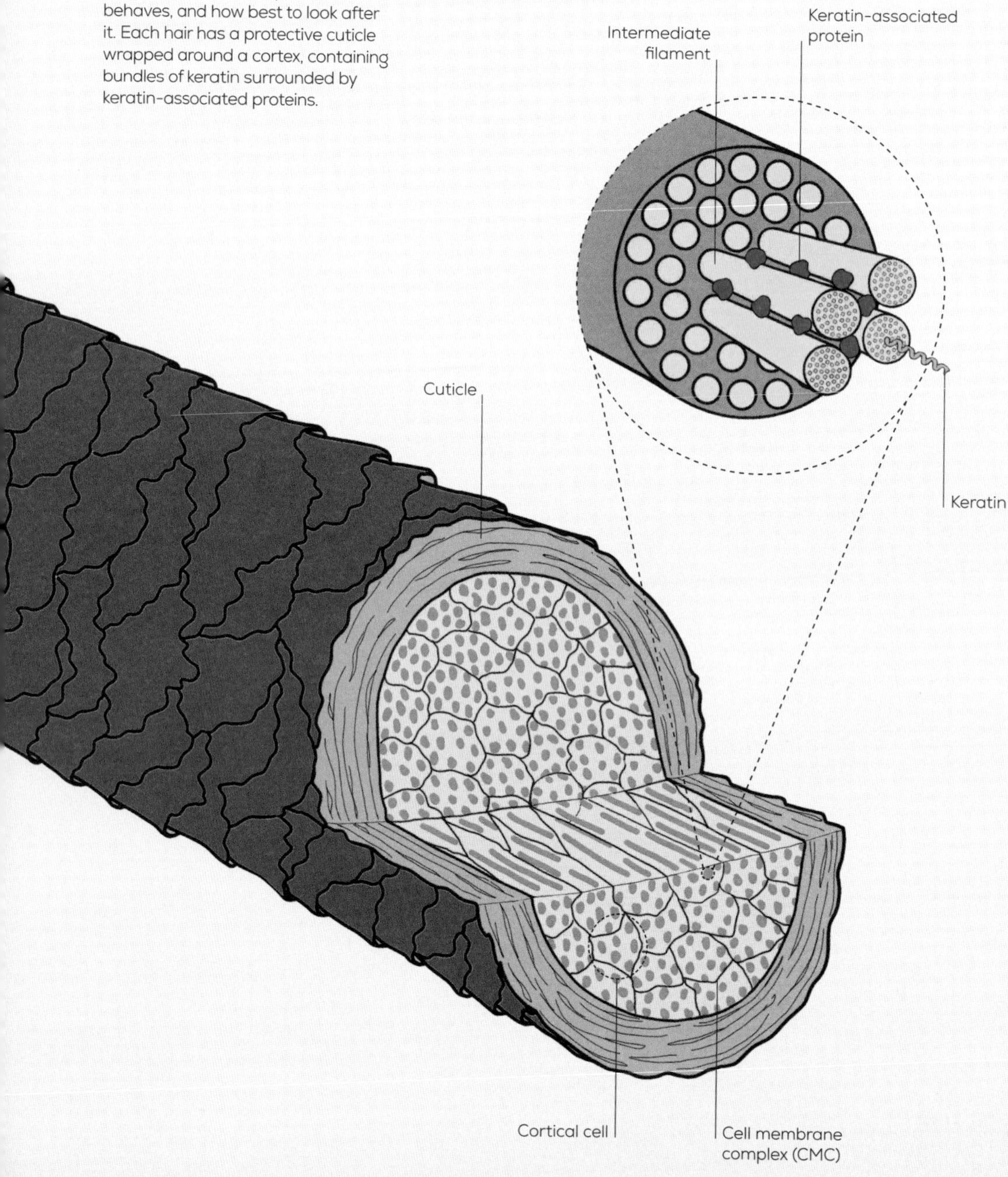

Intermediate filament

Keratin-associated protein

Keratin

Cuticle

Cortical cell

Cell membrane complex (CMC)

What is hair made of?

Human hair is an incredible material that's as strong as steel by weight.

It has an extremely complex structure to achieve this level of strength – some aspects of its structure are still being discovered.

Hair follicle

We have up to 130,000 hairs just on our scalp. Each hair grows from a bulb at the bottom of the hair follicle. In the bulb, matrix cells divide rapidly to produce the cells that make up the hair strand. As the cells travel towards the surface, they die, lose water, and harden. Around 1 cm (½in) of hair is produced each month.

Cuticle

Hair is mostly made of protein, arranged into a thin protective cuticle wrapped around a central cortex.

The cuticle is made of 5–10 layers of overlapping scale-like cells arranged like roof tiles, slanting outwards from the root end. This structure helps push dirt and skin flakes out of the follicle, and it's why hair feels smoother from root to tip.

Each cuticle scale has a hard, water-repellent (hydrophobic) upper surface that gradually transitions into a soft, water-loving underbelly. The water resistance comes from the F-layer, a very thin layer of oily lipids chemically bonded to the top of each cuticle cell. The F-layer also makes hair feel smooth and soft. The cell membrane complex (CMC) sits between cuticle cells, acting as a flexible "glue". This structure makes the cuticle strong, but still allows the hair to bend and move without cracking. The cuticle also acts as a barrier to large molecules, but smaller ones (like water) can travel through the CMC and cuticle underside into the cortex.

Cortex

Under the cuticle is the cortex, which represents about 80% of the hair by mass. It contains long cortical cells stuck together by the CMC.

Inside the cells are two types of protein. First, there are long spirals of keratin twisted into rope-like bundles called intermediate filaments. These lie parallel to each other in a highly structured arrangement. They are surrounded by smaller keratin-associated proteins (KAPs or matrix proteins).

Many bonds glue the two types of protein into a strong but flexible network that is responsible for many hair properties, including its shape, strength, and elasticity.

The cortex also contains melanin pigments. Different hair colours have varying quantities of brown-black eumelanin and yellow-red pheomelanin.

In thicker hairs there is sometimes a largely empty region in the centre called the medulla.

What gives hair its shape?

Hair is mostly made of proteins, which are long chains consisting of many amino acids. Bonds form between separate protein chains to create a network that contributes to hair's strength, but also gives each strand its shape.

Permanent bonds

Hair proteins are abundant in cysteine, a sulfur-containing amino acid that can pair up to form strong disulfide bonds between chains. More disulfide bonds create a harder structure that's more resistant to physical forces and chemical attack. They also have a large influence on the hair's permanent shape.

Ionic or salt bonds form between oppositely charged amino acids in hair proteins. For example, the negative charge on glutamic acid is attracted to the positive charge on lysine. Ionic bonds are broken at very acidic or alkaline conditions (pH below 2 or above 12), and can be weakened by water.

Temporary bonds

Hair also contains temporary bonds that break and reform frequently, such as during washing and heat styling. Many temporary hydrogen bonds in hair join nitrogen or oxygen atoms to certain hydrogen atoms. Each hydrogen bond is weaker than a permanent bond, but there are far more hydrogen bonds, so together they contribute significantly to hair's strength when dry.

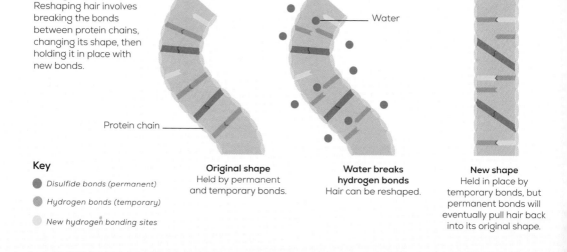

Styling hair
Reshaping hair involves breaking the bonds between protein chains, changing its shape, then holding it in place with new bonds.

Protein chain

Water

Key
- Disulfide bonds (permanent)
- Hydrogen bonds (temporary)
- New hydrogen bonding sites

Original shape
Held by permanent and temporary bonds.

Water breaks hydrogen bonds
Hair can be reshaped.

New shape
Held in place by temporary bonds, but permanent bonds will eventually pull hair back into its original shape.

Hair styling

At a molecular level, hair styling uses heat or water to break temporary bonds, then new bonds are formed to hold the hair's new shape. For example, when curly hair is washed and flat-ironed, the existing hydrogen bonds are broken. The hair is then manipulated into a straighter shape. Drying and cooling creates new temporary bonds which lock the new shape in place. Styling products like hairspray can provide further hold.

Later, when hair is washed, these temporary bonds break. The permanent disulfide and ionic bonds pull hair back into its original curly shape. The temporary bonds also break over time, and with humidity.

Straight versus curly hair

While hair shape can be explained by bonding, why hair is straight or curly in the first place is less clear. Multiple factors seem to contribute to curly hair. The main influence is thought to be asymmetric distributions of cells and proteins across each strand.

Race and hair

The chemical composition of hair doesn't differ much with race, but hair shape (determined by genetics) and cultural practices can have a big impact. Asian hair tends to be straight with a round cross-section, while African hair tends to be curly, with an elliptical cross-section, and European hair tends to lie in between, but there is much variation within any of these very broad groups. African hair tends to be the most fragile, due to its shape and variability along the fibre, leading to points of concentrated stress. Work is ongoing to better understand different hair types and the influence of race and shape on hair properties.

How curly hair forms
Curly hair grows with asymmetric protein density across each hair strand, which causes the hair to curl after it exits the follicle and dries.

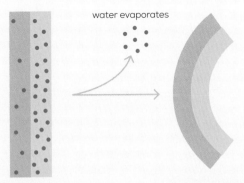

water evaporates

Inside follicle
Curly hair is straight inside the hair follicle, but there is denser protein on one side.

Outside follicle
This causes one side of the hair to shrink more as it exits the follicle and dries, leading to curling.

How does hair become damaged?

Hair is dead once it exits the scalp so it can't repair itself, and both the cuticle and internal cortex begin to accumulate damage.

By the time hair is 14cm (5.5in) long, it has experienced around a year's worth of brushing, washing, drying, and exposure to the elements, as well as any heat styling and chemical treatments you use.

Mechanical damage

Many daily activities can physically damage the hair's surface. Friction from brushes, elastic bands, and even from hair strands rubbing against each other will chip away at the cuticle scales. This leaves a bumpy surface that feels rough, is more prone to tangling, and looks dull as it reflects light unevenly.

Hair's internal structure is also impacted by mechanical stresses from grooming.

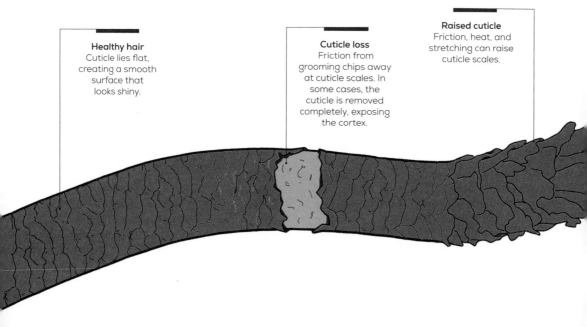

Healthy hair
Cuticle lies flat, creating a smooth surface that looks shiny.

Cuticle loss
Friction from grooming chips away at cuticle scales. In some cases, the cuticle is removed completely, exposing the cortex.

Raised cuticle
Friction, heat, and stretching can raise cuticle scales.

During combing, tangles are pushed to the ends, creating a region with concentrated tugging and bending forces. The ends become particularly rough, and the cuticle may have worn down completely to expose the unprotected cortex.

Mechanical wear and tear happens when hair is dry, but the effects are magnified when wet. Water soaks into hair and breaks hydrogen bonds, making it weaker. The cuticle scales stick up and chip away more easily. Water can also make hair strands stick together, increasing the likelihood of tangling.

However, water can be beneficial for detangling curly and coily hair. The greater number of twists in each strand means strain can be concentrated into particular sections, causing internal cracking. Water can make hair more flexible and loosen its shape, which makes combing easier – this can outweigh the downsides of manipulating hair in its wet, fragile state, although it should still be handled gently to minimize damage.

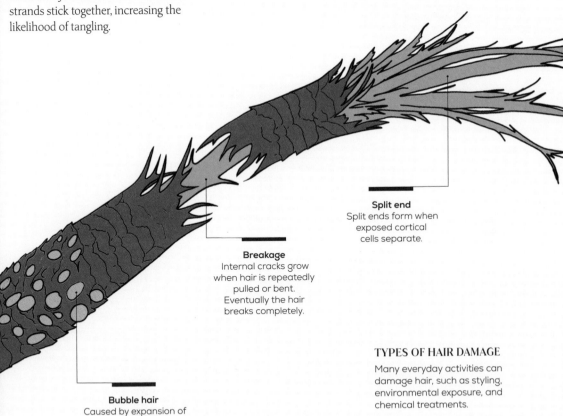

Split end
Split ends form when exposed cortical cells separate.

Breakage
Internal cracks grow when hair is repeatedly pulled or bent. Eventually the hair breaks completely.

Bubble hair
Caused by expansion of water when it boils inside the hair shaft.

TYPES OF HAIR DAMAGE

Many everyday activities can damage hair, such as styling, environmental exposure, and chemical treatments.

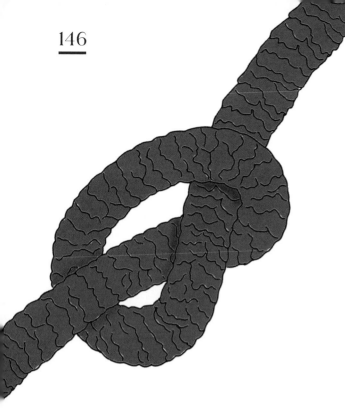

Knot
Texture, friction, movement, and infrequent detangling all contribute to knots.

Oxidation can also remove the oily F-layer from the cuticle's surface, making it rough and dull. It also has higher friction, which increases mechanical damage and tangles. The lipids in the hair's CMC "glue" can also oxidize, weakening the hair's structure. Oxidative damage to hair is accelerated by copper and iron from tap water.

Chemically treated hair absorbs more water, as the F-layer and disulfide bonds are replaced by water-attracting groups. It dries slowly, so hair stays in a fragile state for longer.

The missing F-layer also means damaged hair needs different conditioning ingredients. Uncharged ingredients do not bind well, but positively charged ingredients adhere to damaged regions, which acquire a negative charge – this is exploited when designing products for damaged hair.

Chemical damage

As well as changes in the physical structure of the hair, the chemical composition of its components can also undergo changes (which further impact its physical state).

Oxidation during chemical treatments (perming, chemical straightening, bleaching, oxidative dyeing) can break disulfide bonds. This weakens the hair, and makes the cuticle rougher, thinner, and less compact. Breaking bonds also creates loose protein fragments, which are lost from hair over time.

Heat damage

Heat from hot tools can denature hair's proteins, warping their structures and causing microscopic cracks on the hair surface. Higher temperatures cause more damage. Heat-damaged hair feels rough, and can lose its shape. Dye molecules can break down with heat, leading to colour fade.

Bubble hair can form when hot tools are used on wet hair. Intense heat boils water inside the hair shaft, creating holes as it rapidly expands.

UV damage

UV exposure can cause oxidative damage, weakening the hair structure, degrading specific amino acids, and removing the F-layer. Hair becomes rougher and more fragile. Prolonged UV exposure can also cause colour fade and yellowing.

What's the point of conditioner?

Conditioner might seem like an optional extra that you can skip if you're running late and need to shower quickly, but it can be just as important as shampoo.

While shampoos wash dirt, skin flakes, oil, and styling products from your hair and scalp, conditioners improve the feel and appearance of hair, and protect it against damage.

How conditioners work

Hair conditioners deposit on the hair surface to plug gaps and make it smoother, improving hair's feel and appearance. Conditioners also protect against damage. Smoother strands experience less friction and are less likely to snag. This reduces the mechanical forces during grooming, so the cuticle gets less chipped, and the cortex less cracked. Some conditioners can also block hair dyes from leaching out as quickly, and stick down cuticle scales. Additionally, conditioner lubricates hair while it's wet, and helps it detangle.

Many ingredients are used for conditioning. Almost all hair conditioners contain quats like behentrimonium methosulfate and cetrimonium chloride. These are cationic surfactants similar in structure to cleansing surfactants (see pp58–59), but have a positively charged head. Hair has a negative charge when it's above approximately pH 3.7 (its isoelectric point), such as during washing. The positive heads of the cationic surfactants help them stick to the negatively charged hair to form an oily layer.

Hair conditioners deposit on the surface of hair strands to plug gaps and make them smoother.

When enough cationic surfactants have attached, the hair acquires a slightly positive charge, which repels any more molecules from attaching. This helps the surfactants form a thin layer that feels silky, rather than heavy like oils or sebum. Damaged hair tends to have a more negative charge, so the cationic surfactants will preferentially stick there.

Hair conditioners usually also contain fatty alcohols, which combine with cationic surfactants to create a layered (lamellar) structure. This allows the conditioner to coat hair more easily, and thickens the product texture.

Many other ingredients can be added to conditioners to adjust the properties of the conditioning layer, including cationic polymers, silicones, hydrolyzed proteins,

HOW CONDITIONER WORKS

Conditioners form deposits on hair that smooth it out and protect against further damage.

Undamaged cuticle scales lie flat, and have a slight negative charge.

Undamaged hair
Newer hair has a smoother surface.
This is typical near the roots.

and plant oils. These work primarily on the cuticle, but some ingredients can diffuse inside the hair cortex. Some more durable ingredients can keep hair conditioned through multiple washes.

Do I need conditioner?

Longer hair usually needs hair conditioner since it's sustained more damage. Chemical treatments cause a lot of damage to hair, so it can be very fragile unless conditioned. However, short hair might not need a separate conditioner. Most modern shampoos are "2-in-1" formulas that use polymers or silicones to lightly condition hair, which can be enough to prevent tangling and stop hair from feeling too "squeaky clean".

Damaged cuticle scales are jagged, and become more negatively charged.

Positively charged ingredients are attracted to the more negative damaged regions.

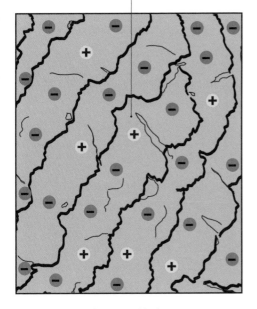

Damaged hair
Grooming, washing, sun exposure, and chemical treatments abrade the cuticle over time.

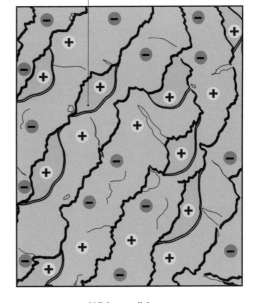

With conditioner
Conditioning ingredients deposit on the surface of the cuticle.

How often should I wash my hair?

Sebaceous glands inside hair follicles produce sebum, which keeps your scalp and hair soft, and helps repel water. However, too much can stick hair together and make it greasy and limp.

Shampoos wash sebum, dirt, skin flakes, and styling products from your hair and scalp. Shampoos are formulated much like other cleansing products. Anionic surfactants (sulfates, sarcosinates, taurates, and isethionates) or non-ionic glucosides are usually the active cleaning ingredients. These disperse oily substances in water, allowing them to be rinsed away efficiently. Non-ionic and amphoteric surfactants boost foam and mildness. Conditioning polymers or silicones are included to reduce tangling and improve hair feel.

Why should I wash my hair?

Many people find that their scalp becomes irritated when they don't wash it regularly, especially if they sweat or use styling products. Sebum, skin flakes, and hair products can build up on the scalp and change the microbial environment. This can cause irritation and inflammation, and contribute to dandruff and malodour. It can also impact hair follicles and interfere with hair growth.

Can I wash my hair too much?

When hair is wet, it's at its most fragile. The outer cuticle repels water, but it can easily

Effects of water on hair
When hair is wet, cuticle scales are raised and more susceptible to damage.

Water-repellent outer scale

Water-absorbent inner scale

Water-absorbent cell membrane complex

Dry hair
Structure is compact, and cuticle scales lie flat along the surface.

pass between cuticle scales. Undamaged hair can absorb up to 30% of its own weight in water, causing it to swell and become 15% thicker in minutes. Damaged hair swells even more.

The reason hair absorbs water so well is its ability to form many hydrogen bonds. When dry, hair proteins form hydrogen bonds with each other to create a strong reinforced network. When wet, the proteins form hydrogen bonds with water instead. This breaks the reinforcements and reduces structural integrity by up to one-third, so wet hair is much more likely to stretch past its breaking point. The cuticle scales are also weakened and lifted, so they break off more easily when rubbed.

An unsuitable shampoo can irritate your scalp, and frequent washing can shorten the effects of hair treatments and remove dyes.

Because of these competing considerations, it's best to wash your hair as often as needed to remove build-up and minimize irritation. Just make sure you handle your hair carefully when wet.

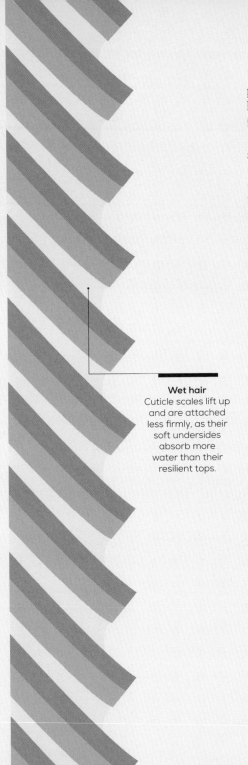

Wet hair
Cuticle scales lift up and are attached less firmly, as their soft undersides absorb more water than their resilient tops.

BEAUTY MYTHS

OIL TRAINING YOUR HAIR
It's commonly thought that if you stop washing your hair, the oil levels will balance out and you won't need to wash as often. To an extent this is true: many people might be washing their hair more than strictly necessary, and only so much oil can build up on hair. But there's no evidence for a biological feedback loop that tells sebaceous glands to slow down when there's more sebum present. Sebum production is largely controlled by hormones and genetics.

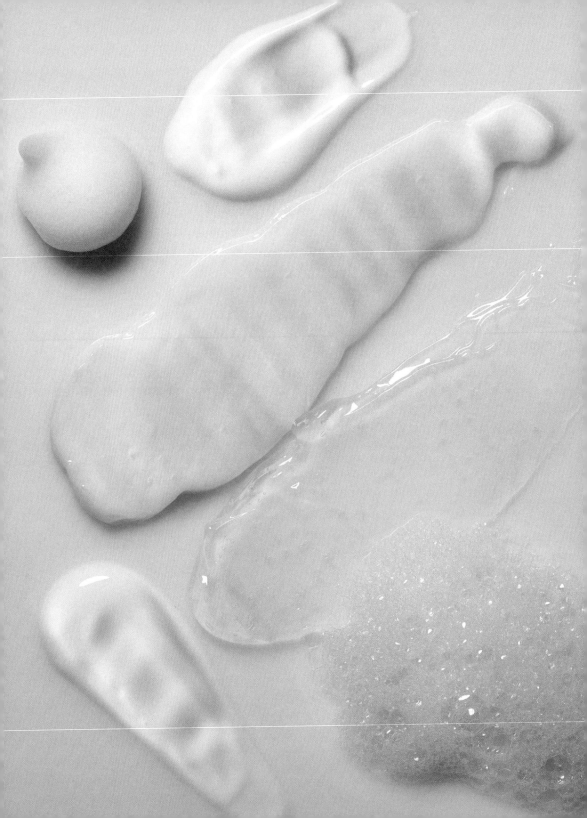

When hair is wet,
it's at its most fragile.
The outer cuticle
repels water, but it can
easily pass between
cuticle scales.

How do I choose shampoo and conditioner?

Hair is extremely diverse, which can make finding an appropriate shampoo and conditioner for your exact hair type very difficult.

Brands use many categories to describe the hair type they're targeting:
Amount of oil: dry versus oily.
Amount or type of damage: chemically treated, dull, long, frizzy, porous.
Thickness of strands: fine versus coarse.
Density of hair: thin versus thick.
Shape (texture): straight, wavy, curly, coily.
Colour: blonde, dark, grey, dyed.
Special considerations: dandruff, 2-in-1, UV protection.
Your hair probably falls into multiple categories offered by the one brand. Additionally, how well a product works can depend on many factors, like how often you wash, how you use the product, what other products you're using, and your hair's exposure to the environment.

Product selection

A good starting point is to choose products formulated for your hair's most pressing need. Additionally, read reviews from people with similar hair to you, and see if you can try a sample.

Conditioning is a balancing act. A thicker conditioning layer leads to lower friction, softer feel, and shinier appearance, but can also weigh hair down and decrease volume. To avoid this, try only conditioning the hair below your ears, and skip conditioning the relatively undamaged roots. This also avoids build-up of conditioner residue on the scalp. While it isn't strictly necessary to use matching shampoo and conditioner, they are often intended to work together. For

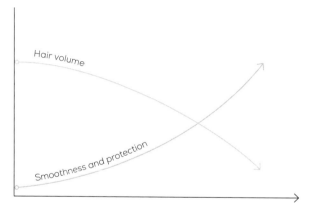

Hair volume

Smoothness and protection

More conditioner deposited

Amount of conditioner
As more conditioner deposits, hair becomes smoother and more protected, but has less volume.

example, a shampoo that deposits a lot of a conditioning polymer might be paired with a lighter conditioner to achieve a particular level of overall conditioning. For long hair, try selecting a shampoo that addresses your scalp's needs, and a conditioner that targets the lengths of your hair.

Should I rotate hair products?

It can be beneficial to switch between products, depending on your hair needs. For example, a clarifying or anti-dandruff shampoo might only need to be used occasionally.

Thickness of strands
The thickness of each individual hair strand determines whether you have coarse or fine hair.

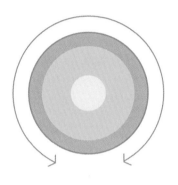 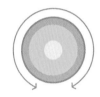

Coarse   Fine

Density of hair
Hair density refers to how close individual hair strands are on the scalp.

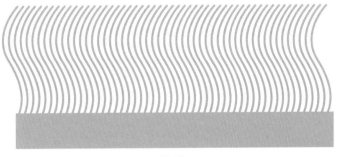

Thick

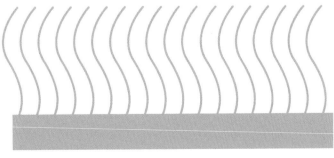

Thin

Why do different hair types need different products?

While the main ingredients used in haircare products are similar, formulas are tweaked to make them more suitable for different hair types.

2-in-1 shampoos are usually designed for hair that doesn't need a separate conditioner. However, most modern shampoos are technically 2-in-1, with conditioning ingredients to prevent tangling during washing and make hair feel less rough. **Medicated shampoos** contain active ingredients to treat conditions like dandruff, lice, and psoriasis. **Baby shampoos** are mild cleansers and do not sting eyes as much.

"Hydrating" products

Unlike skin, adding water to hair usually isn't beneficial. Hair that we consider "hydrated" generally has well-aligned strands, with a smooth, well-conditioned surface. But water has the opposite effect on hair – it often makes it feel rough and limp. In lab experiments, hair that consumers thought felt "more hydrated" actually had lower water content. However, too little water can lead to brittleness and static build-up.

While hair's water content has a big impact on hair's properties, it's difficult to control with products. It quickly adjusts to the surrounding humidity. Water can't be "sealed in" with occlusives like for skin, but a few ingredients like humectants and "bond-builders" may have an effect.

Most modern shampoos are technically 2-in-1, with conditioning ingredients.

HAIR TYPE	PRODUCT FEATURES
Fine or thinning hair	Volumizing products may contain polymers or particles that create structure, and lighter conditioning ingredients to avoid weighing hair down.
Frizzy hair	Ingredients like polymers and emollients can smooth and define hair, while providing humidity resistance.
Chemically treated hair	Higher levels of cationic (positive) conditioning ingredients are needed to adequately condition chemically treated hair, due to its water-loving surface. Speciality ingredients like proteins can also help restore hair properties.
Oily hair	Shampoos formulated for oily hair have greater cleaning power, and leave less conditioning ingredients behind.
Textured hair	Textured hair is more prone to mechanical damage, so it requires highly conditioning products that can reduce friction and improve manageability. However, heavy conditioning can weigh down fine hair and make it lose its shape. Products for textured hair often contain polymers that help define waves, curls, and coils.
Coloured hair	Colour protection shampoos are designed to strip dye from hair less, while conditioners sometimes leave longer-lasting deposits that block dye molecules from leaching out as easily. Metal-chelating ingredients are sometimes included to trap copper ions from tap water, which would otherwise speed up UV-induced pigment changes.
Blonde and grey hair	Shampoos for blonde and grey hair often deposit purple dyes to cancel out the appearance of yellow tones.

What are the benefits of different hair products?

There are many categories of hair products beyond shampoo and conditioner. Here's a guide to some of the most common ones.

Dry shampoos contain starch or silica, which absorb oil then are brushed away. They cannot entirely replace rinse-off shampoos since they do not remove as many substances, and can contribute to build-up. However, they are useful for removing some oil and restoring volume between washes. They come in sprays or shakers.

Co-washing or "no-poo" products use conditioner ingredients (cationic surfactants and fatty alcohols) to wash the hair and scalp. These tend to have poorer cleansing ability and can contribute to scalp build-up over time.

Shampoo bars are made with minimal water and are convenient for travel, but their formulations are more limited and may not be suitable for some hair types. They can potentially have a lower environmental

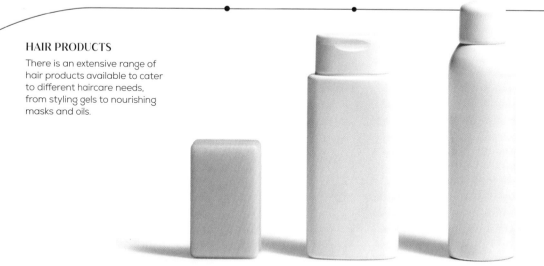

HAIR PRODUCTS

There is an extensive range of hair products available to cater to different haircare needs, from styling gels to nourishing masks and oils.

Shampoo bars
Minimal packaging cleansing product.

Co-washing products
Less cleansing formulas used in place of traditional shampoos.

Dry shampoos
Revive hair between washes by absorbing oil.

impact as less weight needs to be transported, and there is usually less packaging. However, water consumption during use is often the largest contributor to environmental impact for shampoos, so if they take longer to use, any savings might be lost.

Conditioning masks contain similar ingredients to regular conditioners, and essentially do the same task: they leave a protective conditioning layer that makes hair softer, smoother, and shinier. However, they are intended to deliver a higher level of conditioning and are applied for longer. Leaving a regular conditioner for longer can produce a similar effect. They are usually thicker, which makes them easier to use.

Leave-in conditioners also have similar ingredients to regular conditioners, but do not need rinsing and can be used between washes. They come in many forms like sprays, serums, and creams, and are often marketed based on a specific conditioning benefit (e.g. shine, detangling, anti-frizz) but generally provide other common conditioning benefits too.

Hair oils act as leave-in conditioners that add shine, and condition the hair and scalp. These are often pure plant oils. Coconut oil is particularly beneficial, as its narrower structure absorbs slightly into the cortex to replace lost lipids and improve elasticity. However, pure plant oils can be unpleasantly heavy and sticky. Commercial hair oils dilute plant oils or silicones in a base that helps them spread on hair, then evaporates to avoid weighing hair down.

Protein treatments aim to add proteins back into damaged hair to restore some of its properties. The proteins can come from

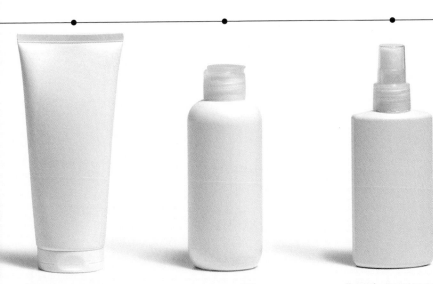

Conditioning masks
Intense conditioning treatments that leave a protective layer behind.

Leave-in conditioners
Conditioners that don't need rinsing.

Protein treatments
Restore damaged hair.

various sources (e.g. wheat, silk) and are often broken into smaller fragments (hydrolyzed). The exact effects depend on the type and size of the proteins, their ability to stick to hair, and the level of hair damage. Some small proteins can penetrate into the cortex to add strength and flexibility, while larger proteins stay on the surface and soften or thicken hair strands.

Bond-building treatments increase bonds inside the cortex to improve its strength. This is not a well-defined category, and many ingredients can be argued to be "bond builders". Some claim to work by linking broken disulfide bonds, while others sit in the hair and block water from breaking hydrogen bonds, or create new hydrogen bonds. They are generally more beneficial for damaged hair, and are often used during or after chemical treatments.

Heat protectants create a thin coating on hair that distributes heat from styling tools more evenly, preventing "hot spots" that receive extremely damaging levels of heat. Many ingredients can create heat-protective films, including silicones and polymers.

UV-protective products generally use sunscreen ingredients to absorb UV before it reaches the hair. This prevents UV-induced oxidative changes, particularly colour changes.

Styling products work by sticking hairs together where they touch, much like welding together pieces of metal. They can

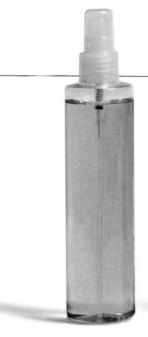

Hair oils
A type of leave-in conditioner to nourish hair.

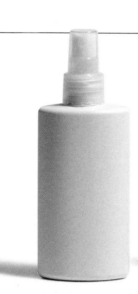

Heat protectants
Leave a thin coating on hair to prevent "hot spots" when styling with heat.

UV-protective products
Use sunscreen ingredients to protect hair from UV damage.

also coat sections of hair in a film that adds rigidity or reduces movement. A huge range of ingredients are used to give different levels of hold and flexibility. Hairsprays, mousses, and gels contain polymers that form a film after the solvent (usually water or alcohol) evaporates. Oil-based styling waxes and creams work similarly but do not dry, so they usually have less hold but allow easy restyling. Styling products help hair resist frizz and humidity by using ingredients that are less affected by water. Many styling products also give other benefits like shine, conditioning, and heat protection. **Volumizing and texturizing products** deposit grippy polymers or particles to increase friction between hair strands.

These are usually applied at the roots and allow hairs to lean on each other to create volume. Sea salt sprays work in a similar way.

Styling products work by sticking hairs together where they touch, much like welding together pieces of metal.

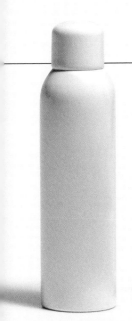

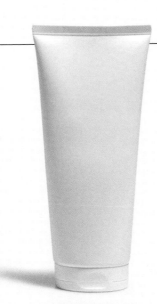

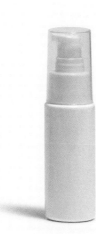

Bond-building treatments
Strengthening treatment for damaged hair.

Styling products
Used to manipulate hair into different styles and to reduce frizz.

Volumizing and texturizing products
Leave deposits in hair to create volume.

Should I avoid particular haircare ingredients?

There are many ingredients that you may be told to avoid in haircare products, but there's usually little truth to these claims.

Myths about the health impacts of these ingredients are fuelled by misinformation, and may be perpetuated in order to sell "free-from" products. The scientific evidence shows that our products are usually very safe.

Sulfates

"Sulfates" usually refers to sodium lauryl sulfate (SLS) and sodium laureth sulfate (SLES), popular cleansing surfactants used in shampoos and skin cleansers. They are commonly thought to be more stripping and drying to hair and skin than other surfactants. This is true for SLS when used alone, but isn't necessarily the case in finished products. Surfactants work in a coordinated way, so the other ingredients and overall formula are crucial in determining how sulfates interact with your hair and scalp. Additionally, SLES is less stripping than many alternative surfactants.

For dyed hair, studies have found that sulfate-containing shampoos can strip less colour than sulfate-free formulas. Additionally, simply washing with water makes a far bigger difference than the product you use, so a sulfate-containing shampoo that allows you to wash less often would be beneficial.

Sulfates sometimes contain contaminants (nitrosamines and 1,4-dioxane) that can cause cancer at high doses. However, they are controlled to a safe level in cosmetic products.

Hair dyes

Para-phenylenediamine (PPD) is used in permanent hair dyes, and can cause allergic reactions. Conduct a skin sensitivity test according to the product instructions before using permanent dyes. Use gloves when applying, and minimize contact with the scalp. Para-toluenediamine (PTD) is a related compound that can also cause reactions if you are allergic to PPD.

In the past, there were concerns about permanent hair dyes causing cancer, based on animal studies and industrial exposures to hair dye ingredients. However, several large-scale reviews have since concluded that hair dye use is not associated with increased cancer risk.

Silicones

Silicone ingredients are used to give hair a smooth feel and shiny appearance, but it's often believed that they weigh hair down. While this can happen when an intensely conditioning product is used on fine hair, many other conditioning ingredients can have this effect, and many silicones are very light in texture.

For example, cyclopentasiloxane evaporates quickly after application, so it can't weigh down hair. Many people avoid "dimethicone" due to its perceived heaviness, but the same name is used for many different dimethicones, which range from very light to very heavy in feel. There are also positively charged silicones like amodimethicone, which stop depositing once the hair's charge is neutralized.

Formaldehyde

Some preservatives like DMDM hydantoin release very small amounts of formaldehyde to kill microbes. These are considered safe as they do not add significantly to our daily formaldehyde exposure from other sources like furniture and food.

However, some "keratin" hair straightening treatments are dangerous. Intense heat during these treatments releases a large amount of formaldehyde gas. Inhaling high doses can cause eye and throat irritation, headaches, and cancers, and is especially dangerous for salon workers. Avoid straightening treatments containing formaldehyde, which may also be labelled as methylene glycol or formalin.

How do bleach and dyes work?

Bleach and dye are common ways of changing your hair colour.

Hair's natural colour comes from melanin, which sits in melanosome granules near the outside of the cortex.

Bleach

Bleaching removes colour by breaking up melanin with hydrogen peroxide and persulfates. A high pH alkaline formula loosens the cuticle, so bleach can diffuse faster into the cortex and access the melanin. Both the bleach and alkali are very damaging to hair. Incomplete destruction of melanin leads to orange or yellow tones, which can be covered with dye.

Direct dyes (temporary and semi-permanent)

Direct dyes contain dye molecules in their final form, and no oxidizing agent. Since melanin is not removed, they don't show up well on darker hair.

Temporary dyes have large coloured molecules that bind weakly to the cuticle, and are removed after a few washes.

Semi-permanent dyes are similar, but may contain smaller dyes that penetrate into the cuticle slightly or adhere to hair more strongly, so they last longer. A slightly alkaline pH is sometimes used to loosen the cuticle for better absorption.

"Toning" shampoos and conditioners also contain direct dye molecules.

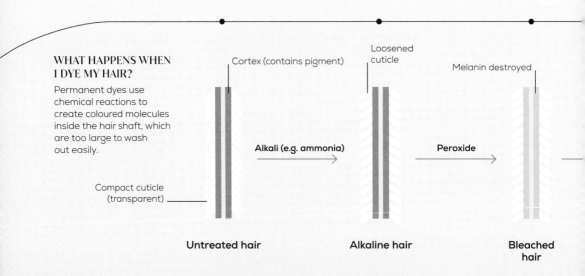

WHAT HAPPENS WHEN I DYE MY HAIR?

Permanent dyes use chemical reactions to create coloured molecules inside the hair shaft, which are too large to wash out easily.

Compact cuticle (transparent)

Cortex (contains pigment)

Alkali (e.g. ammonia)

Loosened cuticle

Peroxide

Melanin destroyed

Untreated hair

Alkaline hair

Bleached hair

Aside from alkaline semi-permanent dyes, direct dyes don't damage hair, and the base is similar to conditioner. However, they can stain hair if the dye is retained too well to be washed out, and bleach may be needed to restore the original colour.

Oxidative dyes (permanent and demi-permanent)

Oxidative dyes contain small precursors that join to form larger coloured molecules after entering the hair shaft.

Immediately before application, a highly alkaline solution containing the precursors is mixed with a hydrogen peroxide developer. The alkali loosens the cuticle, allowing the precursors to penetrate further. Peroxide joins the precursors and decomposes some melanin.

The dye molecules are too large and too deep within the shaft to be washed out, and typically grow out with the hair.

Demi-permanent dyes use weaker alkaline and peroxide solutions that do not loosen the cuticle or lighten melanin as much. The colour washes out faster and less of a colour change is possible, but they are less damaging than permanent dyes.

Henna

Henna leaves are mixed with acid to release lawsone, which reacts with hair proteins to create a permanent reddish-brown colour. There is no bleach or alkali so there is minimal damage, but henna can make it more difficult to perm or dye hair. Some henna products contain metal salts, which can react badly with other hair treatments.

Porosity

Porosity refers to how easily hair absorbs water and treatments. It can greatly affect damage potential and product performance, so radical colour changes are best handled by a professional who can adjust product strength and monitor progress. A strand test is recommended before colouring.

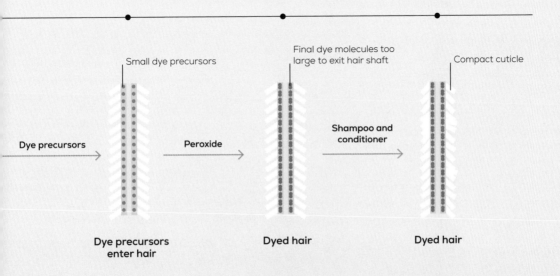

Small dye precursors

Final dye molecules too large to exit hair shaft

Compact cuticle

Dye precursors

Peroxide

Shampoo and conditioner

Dye precursors enter hair

Dyed hair

Dyed hair

How do perming and straightening work?

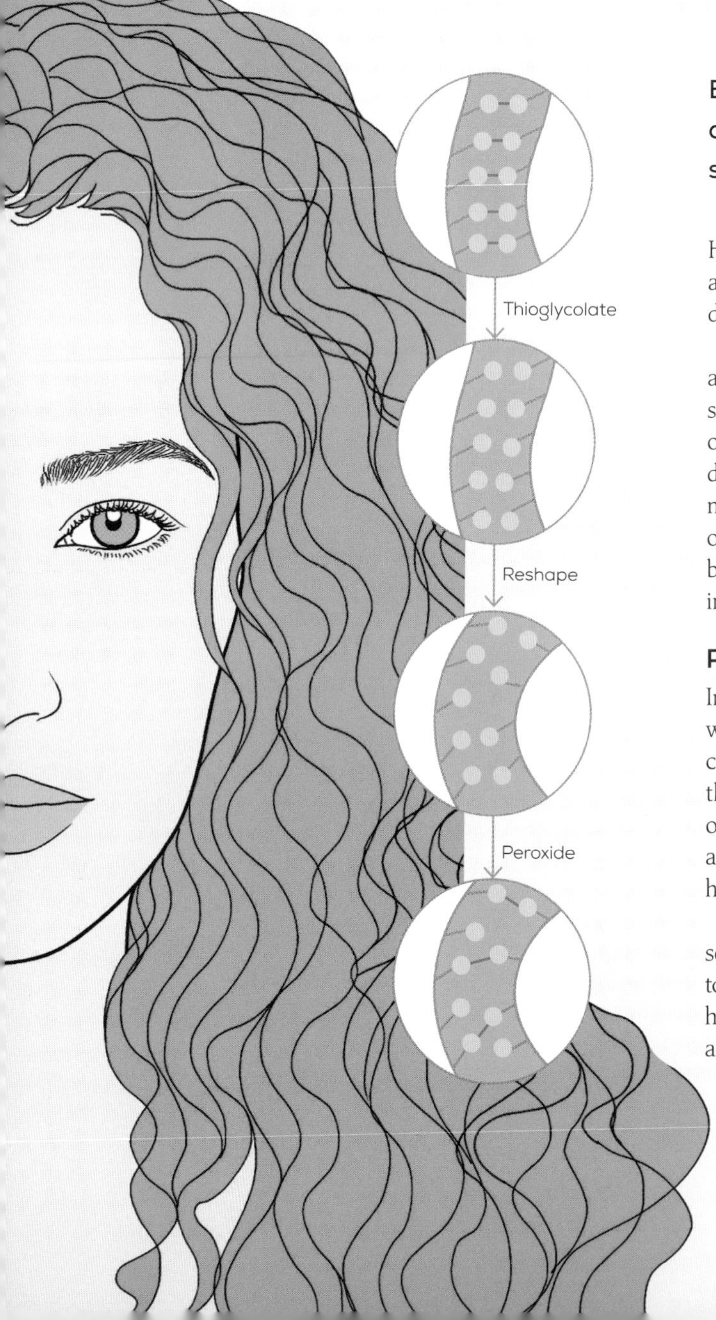

Bonds are vital to hair – they are responsible for not only its strength, but also its shape.

Hair is mostly made of proteins, held in a particular shape by bonds: primarily disulfide, ionic, and hydrogen bonds.

Hydrogen bonds are regularly broken and reformed by water and heat, like during styling. However, the "permanent" shape of hair is determined by the more durable disulfide and ionic bonds, which are far more difficult to break. Permanent curling or straightening involves breaking these bonds and reforming them to hold hair in a new shape.

Perming

In permanent waving (perming), hair is wound around rods to establish the new curl pattern. A reducing agent (usually thioglycolate) is then applied to break some of the disulfide bonds. Next, disulfide bonds are reformed using hydrogen peroxide to hold the new shape.

Some disulfide bonds take longer to form, so hair should not be washed for a few days to ensure remaining bonds are formed in the hair's new shape. Not all the disulfide bonds are reformed, so permed hair is weaker.

Thioglycolate

Reshape

Peroxide

Perming
The structure of hair is altered by breaking disulfide bonds then reforming them in a new pattern, creating curls or waves.

Permanent straightening

Japanese straightening (thermal reconditioning) uses thioglycolate, like perming. However, it is more difficult to straighten hair than to curl it, so hair is rinsed, blow-dried, and flat-ironed before hydrogen peroxide or sodium bromate is applied. Hair should be kept dry and straight for a few days afterwards as new bonds keep forming. As with permed hair, straightened hair is weaker as not all the broken bonds are reformed.

Relaxers are often used to straighten textured African hair, often due to societal pressures and Eurocentric beauty standards, as well as preference or for easier management. Disulfide bonds are broken with highly alkaline hydroxides. Keratin in the cortex changes shape dramatically, and thioether bonds form. Hair is weaker as bonds are missing, but its straighter shape can reduce breakage.

Brazilian keratin treatments make hair straighter and easier to manage, but some curl usually remains. These form new bonds (crosslinks) between hair proteins. The original shape gradually returns over a few months as the crosslinks break. In the original version, formaldehyde and keratin proteins were applied to hair, followed by drying and flat-ironing at 230°C (446°F). The heat caused formaldehyde to crosslink hair proteins. However, this was dangerous, as large amounts of formaldehyde gas could be inhaled (see p163).

Newer "formaldehyde-free" versions use alternative ingredients, but some can still release dangerous amounts of formaldehyde.

Straightening
Permanent straightening uses chemicals to rearrange hair bonds. Some techniques also use hot tools to set the straight shape.

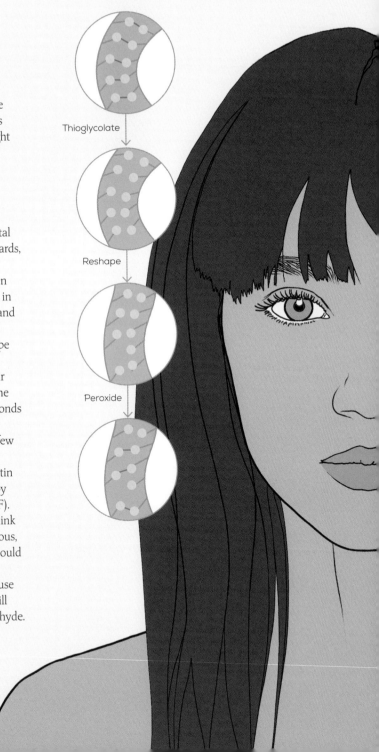

Thioglycolate

Reshape

Peroxide

How do I prevent damage to my hair?

While some hair damage is inevitable, there are many things we can do to keep our hair in the best possible condition.

Detangle
Detangle hair before wetting, or afterwards with conditioner. Hair is more prone to tangling during shampooing. Don't pile hair onto your head – this can tangle it further.

Reduce force
Detangle straighter hair when dry, and curly hair when wet – whichever one requires less force. Handle hair very gently when wet, and don't sleep on wet hair.

WASHING AND CONDITIONING

Condition
Adequate conditioning makes hair smoother, which reduces friction when detangling and styling.

Soften your water
Consider installing a filter if you have hard water, which can reduce the effectiveness of shampoos and conditioners, and impact hair feel.

BEAUTY MYTHS

THE BEST METHOD FOR DRYING HAIR

The amount of hair damage from different drying methods depends a lot on technique. Air drying may not be the least damaging method, as hair remains fragile when wet. A combination of air drying, gently squeezing hair with an absorbent microfibre towel, and using a hair dryer at low heat will minimize damage. In one study, using a hair dryer at a distance of 15 cm (6 in) with continuous motion, resulting in an average hair temperature of 47 °C (116 °F), led to less overall damage than leaving hair to air dry.

Only use very hot tools on dry hair
Intense heat turns water inside hair to steam, which causes "bubble hair" as it expands and damages hair from the inside out.

Prevent knots
Regularly detangle hair to stop knots from building up. Start by brushing out the ends to avoid pushing tangles together, which mats hair further and causes breakages. If you have long hair that gets tangled when you sleep, try plaiting it before bed.

Use hot tools at lower temperatures
Use the lowest temperature possible that achieves the style. Look for tools designed to distribute heat more evenly.

Allow heat protectants to dry before heat styling
These products cannot prevent all damage, but they do distribute heat more evenly and prevent hot spots. Formulas with less water and more alcohol can also reduce the risk of "bubble hair".

GROOMING AND STYLING

Trim hair regularly
Removing rough split ends reduces further damage to hair from friction, tangles, and continued splitting up the hair fibre.

Limit harsh chemical treatments
Bleach, oxidative dyes, perms, and relaxers use harsh alkaline and oxidizing conditions to access the hair cortex, which cause a lot of damage. An experienced professional can tailor the treatment to limit damage, while still achieving a good result.

Protect against sunlight and chlorine
Use hats and UV-protective hair products, and wear swimming caps in pools.

Don't brush your hair too much
Your hair won't grow faster, but it increases damage and breakage.

Check hair tools for jagged edges and cracks
Look for materials that tug less on hair, like ceramic and titanium hot tools. Even switching to hair ties and pillow cases with smoother textures can help reduce breakage.

How do I prevent frizz and flyaways?

Frizz and flyaways are two big reasons for a "bad hair day".

There are several reasons for your misbehaving locks, and a few methods you can use to tame them.

Frizzy hair

Hair looks frizzy when individual hair strands aren't aligned. Split ends, breakage, and layering can contribute to this misalignment. Brushing or combing will align hair, but if the strands are rough, they will quickly pull each other out of alignment again. Conditioning products reduce this by smoothing out hair strands.

The shape of the individual hair strands will also impact alignment and frizziness. Hair strands tend to be more uniform in shape and look less frizzy when you're younger. Hair with more texture is more prone to frizz, so smoothing or straightening treatments will reduce it. Hair can also be temporarily shaped into alignment with heat, and held in place with styling products. However, humidity will cause hair to frizz, as water disrupts the temporary bonds that hold the style and alignment.

Curly or wavy hair looks less frizzy when each piece is "well defined", with many aligned strands with synchronized bends. Wet hair will often assemble into aligned groups when you're detangling, as the surface tension of water pulls strands with similar shapes together. Manipulating the hair too much after it's dried can break up these groups – without water, there is no force to help them realign. To create well-defined hair:

Condition hair thoroughly when wet.
Use styling products like gels and pomades to hold curls together. Anti-humidity products will help control frizz in humid weather.
Use a hair dryer with a diffuser attachment. Minimize brushing and manipulation of hair after drying.

Flyaway hair

Hair loses electrons when rubbed against certain materials like plastics, causing static electricity to build up. Strands become positively charged and repel each other, so some "flyaway" hairs stick out.

Static builds up more easily in dry conditions, since water helps charge dissipate. Some materials have a greater tendency to take electrons from hair and create static. Avoid rubbing hair against objects made of polyester, polyethylene, PVC, and polystyrene. Metals, cotton, wool, and wood tend not to cause static.

Anti-static products contain ingredients like polymers and silicones which reduce friction, so there is less contact between hair and other objects and hence less electron transfer. The conditioning layer can also increase surface conductivity and help disperse static. Styling products like hairsprays and mousses can hold the hair's shape and stick down flyaway strands. Dampening hair with water can also help.

Hair strands
Sleek or frizzy hair, defined curls, and flyaways all come from how individual hair strands are arranged relative to each other.

FRIZZ

Aligned
Smooth hair reflects light evenly

Unaligned
Light isn't reflected evenly, so hair looks frizzy

CURLS ALIGNING

Water in between strands
pulls hair into alignment

FLYAWAYS

Repulsion

Electrons are transferred
to plastic comb

Positively charged hairs
repel and become "flyaways"

Why is my hair falling out?

There are many possible causes of hair loss.

Unlike many species, human hair does not have a noticeable shedding phase. This is because our hair is distributed more evenly at different stages of the growth cycle (see below), so there is a relatively constant shedding of 50–100 hairs a day. There are some seasonal variations: most people have slightly less telogen hairs in spring and slightly more in autumn, when noticeable shedding can occur.

In contrast, many animals have hairs that enter the "dead" telogen phase in a more synchronized manner, shedding their winter coats in spring.

Sudden hair loss

There are many reasons why people can experience hair loss, and causes can overlap. It can indicate an underlying health problem, which may require treatment. Make sure you seek medical attention if you notice unexplained hair loss.

HAIR GROWTH CYCLE

Hair growth occurs in a cycle, roughly divided into three stages.

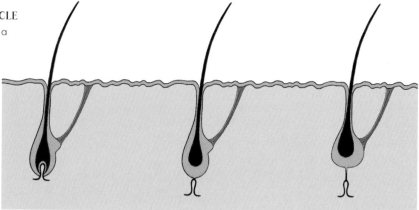

Anagen (growth): around 3 years
New cells are produced in the bulb, causing the hair to lengthen. The duration of anagen determines the maximum hair length.

Catagen (death): around 3 weeks
The bulb dies and detaches from the papilla, which controls growth. It becomes a colourless club, which is pushed upwards as the follicle shortens.

Telogen (rest): around 3 months
The hair strand sheds when we wash or brush our hair, or it can be pushed out as the new hair grows.

Postpartum hair loss During pregnancy, anagen is prolonged leading to thicker hair. Increased shedding and thinner hair are common after childbirth as hormones and hair cycling normalize.

Telogen effluvium Severe emotional or physical stress can cause a large proportion of hair strands to enter telogen in unison. This usually occurs evenly all over the scalp. Common causes include childbirth, severe illness, thyroid disorders, chronic diseases, iron deficiency, and certain medications. Shedding usually occurs a few months after the stress, and often the exact cause is not found. Normal cycling usually resumes 3–6 months after the stress is removed. It can sometimes persist, particularly in middle-aged women.

Chemotherapy Cancer drugs can cause hair to fall out, often accompanied by scalp irritation. Hair usually grows back a couple of months after treatment ends.

Uneven hair loss

Male pattern hair loss (androgenetic alopecia) The most common form of hair loss, affecting about half of men by age 50. It occurs when dihydrotestosterone causes hair follicles to shrink and produce finer, shorter hairs like those found on the body.

Female pattern hair loss A similar condition that affects up to 1 in 3 post-menopausal women. Hair thins from the centre of the scalp towards the sides, with little hairline involvement. The role of hormones is less clear than for male pattern hair loss, but there is a strong genetic component to both.

Alopecia areata Patchy hair loss linked to autoimmune disorders, when the body mistakenly attacks cells in hair follicles. It can progress to the entire scalp or entire body. It proceeds unpredictably and there

is no reliable treatment, but it often reverses spontaneously. Intralesional steroid injections and Janus kinase inhibitors can help.

Traction alopecia Pulling on hair repeatedly can end the growth phase prematurely, and hair loss can be permanent if the pulling continues. Often caused by tight hairstyles.

Scarring or cicatricial alopecias involve the destruction of hair follicles.

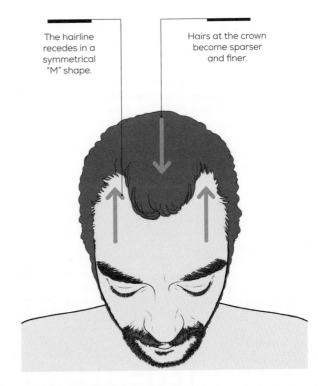

The hairline recedes in a symmetrical "M" shape.

Hairs at the crown become sparser and finer.

Male pattern hair loss
Thinning tends to follow a typical pattern that progresses over time.

How do I reduce dandruff?

Dandruff is a common condition where there is excessive, visible flaking of the scalp and it becomes itchy, dry, red, and inflamed.

WHY DANDRUFF FORMS

There are two main factors that contribute to the formation and symptoms of dandruff.

MALASSEZIA OVERGROWTH

Malassezia yeast is normally found on the scalp, but contributes to dandruff when the microbial balance is disturbed. This is exacerbated by moisture (e.g. from hats) and is more common with oily skin.

More free fatty acids
The yeast feeds on sebum and converts it to free fatty acids.

Leaky barrier
The immature cells form a leakier barrier. Dry weather can exacerbate moisture loss.

INCREASED CELL TURNOVER

Dead cells in the stratum corneum create a protective barrier on the scalp. In dandruff, these cells are produced faster, leading to more dead cells to shed.

Immature cells
Barrier cells do not have enough time to mature before they reach the surface.

Many anti-dandruff shampoos only deposit the active ingredient during rinsing, so shampoo twice for a stronger effect.

Antifungals
Many dandruff treatments kill *Malassezia* yeast, including zinc pyrithione, piroctone olamine, ciclopirox, ketoconazole, and selenium sulfide. These are commonly used in shampoos.

Shampoos
Shampooing regularly keeps yeast and sebum in check. Many anti-dandruff shampoos only deposit the active ingredient during rinsing, so shampoo twice for a stronger effect.

Treatments

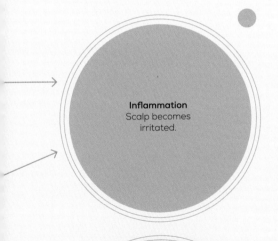

Inflammation
Scalp becomes irritated.

Steroids
Steroids reduce inflammation and normalize cell turnover. Severe dandruff may need oral steroids.

Larger flakes shed
Immature cells do not separate properly, leading to larger flakes.

Coal tar and salicylic acid
Help break up flakes and reduce inflammation. Coal tar also slows cell production.

How can I treat thinning hair?

The first step to treat thinning hair is to try to find the cause. An underlying health condition such as iron deficiency or a thyroid disorder can cause hair loss, and once the condition is managed hair loss stops.

Hair loss can sometimes resolve without treatment. Some medications or procedures can slow or even reverse hair loss.

Treatments and procedures

Minoxidil is used for many types of hair loss. It causes hair to grow thicker and increases the proportion of growing hairs relative to dormant ones. A 2% or 5% liquid or foam is usually applied to the scalp twice daily. It is also used as an oral medication.

Finasteride and dutasteride are oral medications that reduce dihydrotestosterone, making them good treatments for male pattern hair loss. They can also be applied to the scalp.

Minoxidil, finasteride, and dutasteride need to be used continuously to maintain their effect. Once stopped, hair usually returns to the level it would've reached if untreated.

Tretinoin is a common skin treatment, but may stimulate hair growth too.

Prostaglandin analogues like bimatoprost

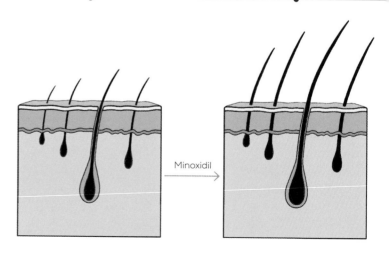

How minoxidil works
Minoxidil is the most common treatment for hair loss. It thickens hair, and shifts more into the anagen phase.

Minoxidil

lengthen and thicken eyelashes by prolonging the anagen phase. However, these are relatively untested for treating the entire scalp and may have side effects.
Anti-androgenic medications may help with female pattern hair loss.
Hair restoration surgery is a very effective option for severe hair loss, but results are highly dependent on the surgeon.
Low level laser therapy (LLLT) uses red light to stimulate hair follicles. While the evidence for its effectiveness is not robust, it is very safe.
Microneedling can be used to wound the scalp in a controlled way, triggering the repair response and activating stem cells in hair follicles. It can also help topical medications absorb. Microneedling is best performed by a professional as low quality and non-sterile devices can cause scarring, infection, and further hair loss.
Platelet-rich plasma (PRP) involves injecting concentrated platelets from blood

into the scalp to stimulate growth and repair. Studies on its efficacy are mixed.
Steroids and topical immunotherapy are used for autoimmune-related hair loss.
Anti-dandruff treatments may help if dandruff is contributing to hair loss, potentially through inflammation.

Disguising hair loss

Hair concealers (particularly those containing fibres) can disguise thinned areas.
Scalp micropigmentation is a form of cosmetic tattooing that mimics stubble.
Cosmetic products can thicken hair strands and add volume. Some active ingredients like caffeine and niacinamide can absorb into hair and thicken individual strands, while polymers and silicones in volumizing products stiffen hairs by coating them. Conditioners that weigh down hair should be avoided.

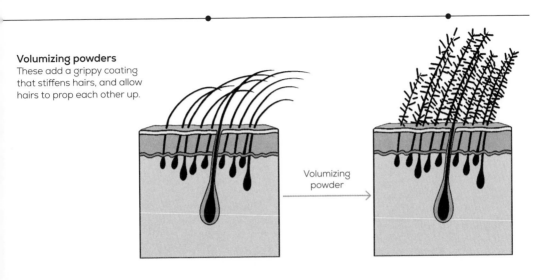

Volumizing powders
These add a grippy coating that stiffens hairs, and allow hairs to prop each other up.

Volumizing powder

Makeup

What are pigments?

Since ancient times, we have used coloured pigments to decorate our faces and bodies. Similar pigments can be found in makeup products today.

Pigments are coloured because they selectively absorb some colours of light. White light contains all the colours in roughly equal amounts. When it hits a pigment, some colours are absorbed, and the remaining colours are reflected into our eyes to create the final colour we perceive.

Pigments in makeup

Pigments are included in makeup as tiny insoluble particles. Multiple pigments are mixed to create different shades. The surfaces of pigment particles are often coated with substances like silicones, silanes, or lecithin to help them resist sweat and smudging. They also blend more smoothly on skin, and keep the product colour and texture more even during manufacture. There are two main categories of pigments: organic and inorganic.

Organic pigments have carbon-based structures similar to organic sunscreen filters, but are larger so they absorb visible wavelengths instead of UV. Most are synthetic. Most organic colours start off as soluble, transparent dyes, which limits their use in makeup. To make them opaque, they are combined with aluminium, barium or calcium compounds to form insoluble "lakes".
Inorganic pigments contain transition metals that absorb coloured light. Many inorganic pigments can be found in nature, but the versions used in makeup are usually manmade to achieve higher purities and more consistent colours.

Effect pigments

Shimmer products contain effect pigments. Different particle sizes and quantities are used to create finishes that range from a subtle satin glow to sparkly glitter.

Organic pigments
These are generally brighter in colour than inorganic pigments, but are less stable and can change colour over time.

Blue 1 lake

Red 6 lake

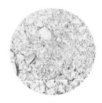

Yellow 5 lake

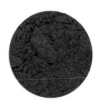

Red 7 lake

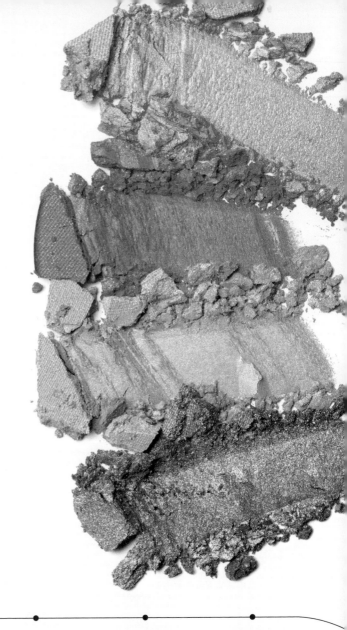

Coloured shimmer comes from using pearlescent pigments that work by interference rather than absorption. Their particles are layered, with multiple reflective surfaces, so light bouncing off them is out of sync. This causes some coloured wavelengths to be intensified (constructive interference), while others are cancelled out (destructive interference).

Single shimmer colours come from synthetic pearl pigments, which consist of very flat particles coated in a uniform transparent layer. The colour produced depends on the thickness of the added layer. The particles are usually mica, fluorphlogopite (synthetic mica) or borosilicate, with a titanium dioxide or iron oxide coating. Absorption pigments can be attached to the particles to create more complex effects.

Subtle rainbow iridescence was originally created using guanine from fish scales or bismuth oxychloride, but synthetic pearl pigments are now more common.

Bright metallic shimmers use metal pigments made from powdered aluminium, bronze or copper.

Inorganic pigments
While these are more stable than organic pigments, their colours are duller. They are the only pigments used in mineral makeup.

Titanium dioxide
TiO_2

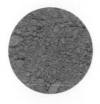

Yellow iron oxide
$FeO(OH) \cdot H_2O$

Red iron oxide
Fe_2O_3

Manganese violet
$NH_4MnP_2O_7$

What are the different types of makeup?

Makeup comes in more forms than any other type of product. It generally contains coloured pigments, dispersed in a base that helps it spread evenly, and last through movement and sweat without smudging or transfer.

Primer
Prepares skin for makeup products. It can moisturize, smooth or illuminate skin, and help makeup adhere better and last longer.

Brow gel and pomade
Hold eyebrow hairs in place. They can be tinted or clear.

Foundation
Skin-coloured product, usually applied to large areas of skin. Foundation with lighter coverage or skincare benefits may be called BB or CC cream, or tinted moisturizer.

Concealer
More opaque than foundation. Used to cover smaller areas like blemishes and dark circles.

Setting powder
Sets liquid and cream products by absorbing oils. Used before powder products to make blending easier. Tinted powder gives some coverage, while translucent powder won't add colour but can blur, mattify, or add glow.

Lip liner
Used to reduce feathering, or alter the lip shape. Can use over the entire lip for longer-lasting colour.

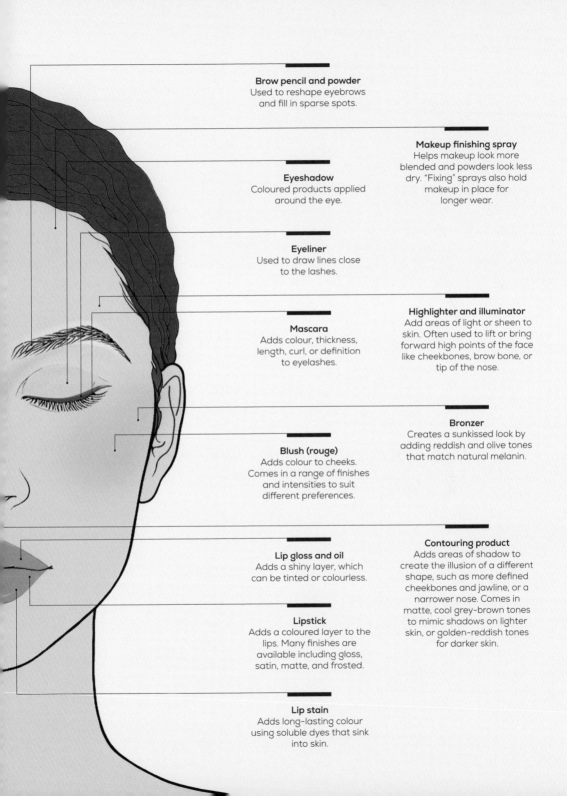

Brow pencil and powder
Used to reshape eyebrows
and fill in sparse spots.

Makeup finishing spray
Helps makeup look more
blended and powders look less
dry. "Fixing" sprays also hold
makeup in place for
longer wear.

Eyeshadow
Coloured products applied
around the eye.

Eyeliner
Used to draw lines close
to the lashes.

Highlighter and illuminator
Add areas of light or sheen to
skin. Often used to lift or bring
forward high points of the face
like cheekbones, brow bone, or
tip of the nose.

Mascara
Adds colour, thickness,
length, curl, or definition
to eyelashes.

Bronzer
Creates a sunkissed look by
adding reddish and olive tones
that match natural melanin.

Blush (rouge)
Adds colour to cheeks.
Comes in a range of finishes
and intensities to suit
different preferences.

Contouring product
Adds areas of shadow to
create the illusion of a different
shape, such as more defined
cheekbones and jawline, or a
narrower nose. Comes in
matte, cool grey-brown tones
to mimic shadows on lighter
skin, or golden-reddish tones
for darker skin.

Lip gloss and oil
Adds a shiny layer, which
can be tinted or colourless.

Lipstick
Adds a coloured layer to the
lips. Many finishes are
available including gloss,
satin, matte, and frosted.

Lip stain
Adds long-lasting colour
using soluble dyes that sink
into skin.

What's in lipstick?

Formulating a makeup product is a balancing act. Lipstick, for example, needs to be hard enough not to break when you apply it, but soft enough to leave a thin layer on your lips.

This layer needs to be uniform in texture and colour, and must be durable – a challenge, since your lips move a lot and are frequently exposed to water. At the same time, it needs to be easily removed at the end of the day.

Base ingredients

Lipstick bases contain mostly oily ingredients, which help repel water.

The proportions are adjusted to give the desired hardness and texture during application, along with the required properties of the final film, like transfer resistance and emolliency.

- Waxes are more solid at room temperature, and make lipsticks harder. Candelilla wax, ozokerite, and microcrystalline wax are most commonly used.
- Oils are liquids that soften the lipstick and add shine, keep colour even, and help the lipstick glide. They also prevent dryness and flaking, since the lips do not produce sebum. They include polybutene, isostearyl isostearate, and castor oil.
- Film formers like polymers can be added to improve transfer resistance.

MAKING LIPSTICK

These steps are used for manufacturing a standard lipstick.

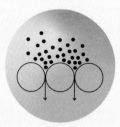

Step 1
Pigments are ground and dispersed in oils and solvents until even.

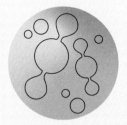

Step 2
Waxy ingredients are melted, then pigment mixture is added and mixed until uniform.

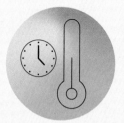

Step 3
Mixture is cooled slightly before adding sensitive ingredients like speciality pigments, antioxidants, and preservatives.

What's wrong with my lipstick?

Beads of oil ("sweating" or syneresis): These form when oils and waxes in the base separate over time.

Fuzzy white spots: These can look like mould but are usually crystals of separated wax or emulsifier, similar to bloom on chocolate.

Pigments

Lipsticks usually contain both insoluble pigments for opacity, and staining colours for longer wear. Pearl pigments are added for shimmer finishes.

Warm-toned red lipsticks often use Red 6 Lake and Red 21, while cool-toned red lipsticks often use Red 7 Lake and Red 27. Colour-change lipsticks darken after application. These usually use Red 27 or 21 and don't give a custom shade based on lip pH as they often claim – these dyes simply turn pink with water.

Bleeding or feathering – when colour travels outside the lips along skin furrows – occurs when pigments are slightly soluble in oils. To prevent feathering, avoid oily, liquid lip products, and apply gloss sparingly, away from the lip edge. Longwear lipsticks feather less. Lip primers and liners can smooth out lines before application.

Other ingredients

Oils in the base can become rancid, so antioxidants are added to slow this down. Flavours and fragrances are important to cover unpleasant smells and tastes.

Skincare ingredients added to lipsticks include UV filters (lips are a common site for skin cancer), peptides, and antioxidants. Instant plumping lipsticks contain irritants like capsicum or ginger extract to temporarily swell up lips, and need to be reapplied to maintain the effect.

Matte lipsticks contain powders like silica or nylon to create a bumpy surface, so reflected light is diffused.

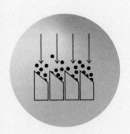

Step 4
Mixture is poured carefully into moulds to reduce pigment settling and air bubbles.

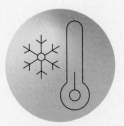

Step 5
Lipsticks are cooled to harden.

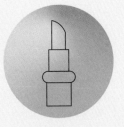

Step 6
Sticks are released from moulds and inserted into tubes.

Step 7
Lipsticks are passed through a flame to melt the surface slightly for a shiny finish.

They also contain less oil, which can make them more drying but longer-wearing.

Lip glosses contain far more oily ingredients for a shinier finish. This gives a liquid texture, so they often come in tubes and are less longwearing.

Longwear lipsticks are usually liquids containing silicone polymers. After application, the solvents evaporate to leave a durable pigmented film. Newer versions come in stick form, with snug packaging.

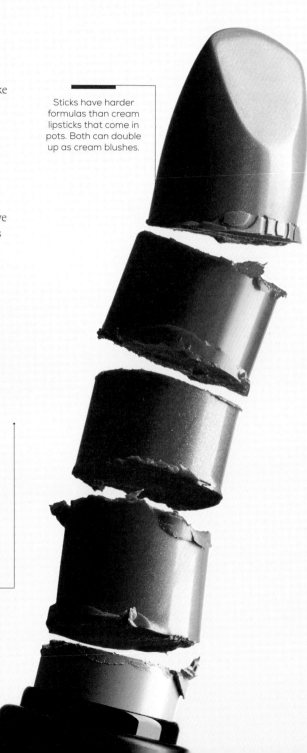

Sticks have harder formulas than cream lipsticks that come in pots. Both can double up as cream blushes.

BEAUTY MYTHS

EATING LIPSTICK
It's been suggested that we eat 3kg (6$\frac{1}{2}$lb) of lipstick over a lifetime. This is a massive overestimate, equating to 800 whole lipsticks! On average, lipstick users apply 24mg a day, or 600g (21oz) over 70 years if applied every single day. The amount eaten is far less – a lot ends up on tissues and cups, and there's still some left on the lips at the end of the day.

What's in a foundation?

Foundations come in many forms: liquids, creams, mousses, sticks, and powders.

Liquid foundation

Almost all liquid foundations are water-in-silicone emulsions, due to their superior properties. When combined with film-forming polymers, they have an unmatched ability to create a durable, flexible, evenly coloured layer on skin. They require minimal skill to apply and dry fast enough to prevent transfer, but slow enough to allow blending.

Emulsions consist of two phases that don't mix (see p30). In water-in-silicone foundations, the continuous phase is based on silicones and contains the ingredients that create the foundation film:

- Pigments are responsible for colour and coverage. Pearl pigments are added for more luminous finishes. Pigment particles are usually surface-treated.
- Silicones and other oily liquids act as solvents to keep the other ingredients mixed together. Some are volatile and evaporate to leave the other components stuck to the skin. Others can also act as moisturizers.
- Film formers create a durable but comfortable film on skin. In longwear foundations, these are usually silicone-based polymers.

Surface-treated particles
Surface treatments allow more uniform makeup formulas, help products blend smoothly, and improve wear on skin.

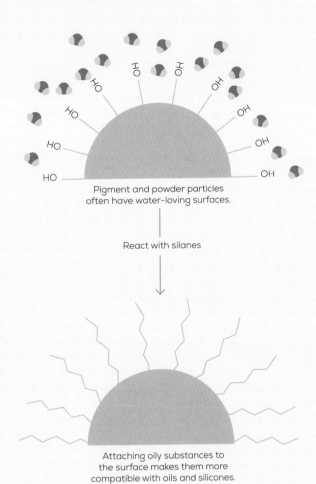

Pigment and powder particles often have water-loving surfaces.

React with silanes

Attaching oily substances to the surface makes them more compatible with oils and silicones.

TYPES OF FOUNDATION

White titanium dioxide is added to increase coverage but can look ashy on darker skin, so zinc oxide is sometimes used instead.

Tinted moisturizers and BB creams have less pigment and contain skincare actives.

Concealers are usually thicker, and have more pigment – up to 40%, while foundations usually have below 10%.

Oil-based cream foundations in pans or jars have similar formulas to sticks.

Two-way powder cakes can also be applied wet for higher coverage.

Powder foundations give buildable coverage, and can be used after setting powder for more coverage.

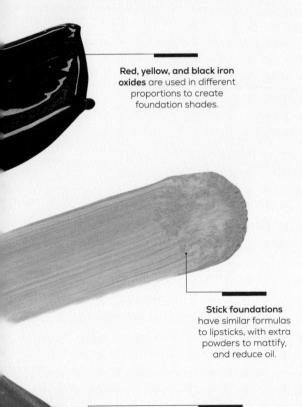

Red, yellow, and black iron oxides are used in different proportions to create foundation shades.

Stick foundations have similar formulas to lipsticks, with extra powders to mattify, and reduce oil.

To make a foundation more luminous, mix in a few drops of liquid illuminator.

- Viscosity modifiers keep pigments from settling and clumping, and thicken the product.
- Powders like silica, mica, or kaolin create a silky texture, absorb oil, and help pigments spread. They can also diffuse light for a soft-focus "HD" effect that makes skin look smoother while remaining natural.
- Oil-soluble skincare ingredients like sunscreens and vitamins can also be added.

The water-based dispersed phase is present as droplets, suspended by emulsifiers. It creates a light feeling upon application, and contains water-soluble skincare ingredients, emulsion stabilizers, and preservatives.

Colour correction

Colour-correcting products neutralize their complementary colours, and are layered under regular foundations and concealers when those don't provide enough coverage on their own. For example, green covers up redness, yellow covers up purple undereye circles, and orange covers up blue-grey stubble and pigment.

HOW DO I FIND THE RIGHT FOUNDATION FOR MY SKIN TONE?

It's best to try out foundations on your face and look at them in natural lighting. Store lighting can distort colours, so check the colour match outside after applying a sample. Some foundations change colour after they dry. This is commonly called "oxidation", but actually comes from the solvent evaporating, or sweat and oil soaking in – much like how wet fabrics can change colour when they dry.

Most people's bodies are a different colour from their faces, due to differences in sun exposure, skin thickness, and skin sensitivity. If you want to take a tip from makeup artists, consider matching your foundation colour to your chest or neck for a more cohesive look.

What goes into powder makeup?

Pure pigments are powders, but do not make good makeup products on their own. People in prehistoric and ancient times used bases like animal fats, oils, or saliva to stick pigments to skin.

In modern powder products, the base consists of powders that dilute the pigments to a suitable intensity, give the right level of slip during application, and absorb oils. They need to be translucent enough to not look ashy, and will contribute to the final finish on skin. Optical blurring powders can be added to improve skin feel and make skin look smoother. Surface treatments and binders help the product spread evenly and adhere to skin.

Pressed powders

Powders can come loose in a jar, or pressed into a pan. Pressed powders require a greater input of binders to keep them stuck together. When pressing, too much pressure makes the cake too hard – the product becomes difficult to pick up, and forms shiny "glazed" patches when rubbed with a brush. Too little pressure makes a soft cake that breaks with small impacts.

Powder tips

Powders usually blend best on top of other powders. Use setting powder over tacky cream and liquid products to create a smooth base and stop powders from sticking.

Use light-diffusing powders with silica sparingly for flash photography – they can show up as stark white patches.

Eyeshadow fallout occurs when loose particles drop onto the cheeks and undereye during application. This tends to happen with larger pearlescent particles, eyeshadows with the wrong mix of binders, or if your brush is overloaded with powder. To prevent fallout from messing up your makeup, you can apply eyeshadow before applying foundation. A thick layer of moisturizer on the undereye area stops stray pigments from staining skin, and can be wiped off easily. Tap the brush on the back of your hand before application to push the powder evenly into the brush, and remove any excess.

Eye primers can reduce fallout and creasing, smooth out application and intensify colours. Many primers contain film-forming polymers to make them sticky.

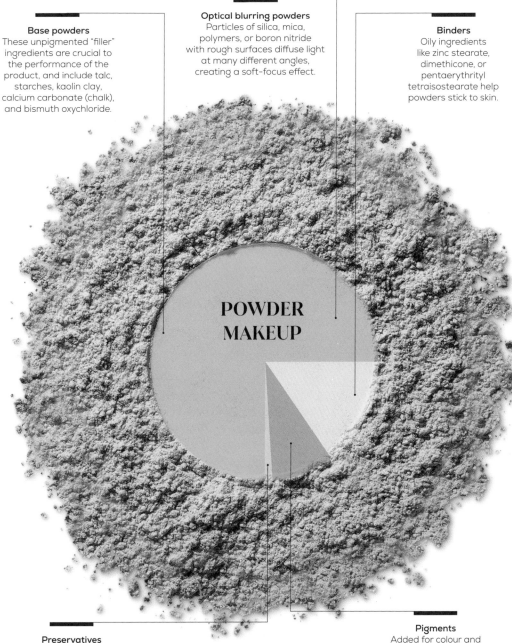

Base powders
These unpigmented "filler" ingredients are crucial to the performance of the product, and include talc, starches, kaolin clay, calcium carbonate (chalk), and bismuth oxychloride.

Optical blurring powders
Particles of silica, mica, polymers, or boron nitride with rough surfaces diffuse light at many different angles, creating a soft-focus effect.

Binders
Oily ingredients like zinc stearate, dimethicone, or pentaerythrityl tetraisostearate help powders stick to skin.

POWDER MAKEUP

Preservatives
Used in powder products that can absorb moisture from the air and support microbial growth.

Pigments
Added for colour and opacity. In shimmer formulas, pigments are often attached to mica particles that also act as the base.

How does mascara work?

Mascaras are one of the top-selling makeup products. They coat the lashes in a film that can add colour, thickness, length, curl, or definition.

Formula

Mascara needs to be thick enough to cover the eyelashes without too many coats, but thin enough to apply easily. The final film needs to be smudgeproof, and flexible enough to resist flaking off.

Black is the most popular shade, and uses black iron oxide or carbon black pigment. Waxes (beeswax, carnauba wax) and powders (silica, clay) make the film thicker for more volume. Film-forming polymers or gums add flexibility, keep the film together, and prevent smudging. Tubing mascaras use a high input of acrylate polymers to create a coating that resists water and flaking, but is easily removed as intact "tubes" with warm water.

Standard water-resistant and tubing mascaras are oil-in-water emulsions. Water helps swell up lashes and form a curl. Emulsifiers help keep it mixed with the oily film-forming ingredients.

Waterproof mascaras are usually water-in-oil emulsions, and contain more oily ingredients. Isododecane is often used as the solvent, and evaporates quickly after application to prevent smudging.

Since mascara is applied close to the eye, there is a high risk of infection if it is contaminated. Preservatives are used even in water-free mascaras.

Special mascaras

Lengthening mascaras contain tiny nylon or rayon fibres that stick to the ends of lashes.

Tubing mascaras resist water, smudging, and flaking, but are easily removed. They tend to be good at separating and lengthening lashes, but usually thicken and curl less than traditional mascaras.

Two-step products have two mascaras designed for different benefits – for example, the first step might be volumizing while the second is lengthening. A similar effect can be achieved by using a second mascara after the first one dries.

Tips

If a mascara doesn't work well, it might apply better with a different, disposable wand. To reduce clumping, wipe excess product off the brush with a tissue before applying. A lash comb can separate clumps.

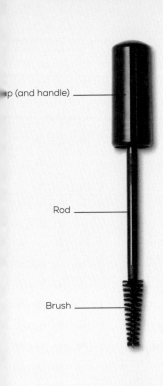

Cap (and handle) —

Rod —

Brush —

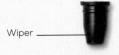

Wiper —

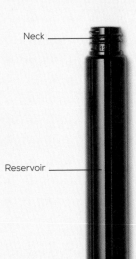

Neck —

Reservoir —

DOES THE BRUSH MATTER?

Yes! The brush has a big impact on how the mascara applies. Different applicators will change film thickness, smoothness, and lash separation.

1 Straight mascara brushes are the most common.

2 and **3** Curved and hourglass wands can reach more lashes in one swipe for more even application.

4 Thinner brushes are good for applying to the base of the lashes and lower lashes, and can achieve a more natural look on sparser lashes.

5 and **6** Tapered brushes add volume quickly, while allowing precise application using the narrower tip.

7 Ball tips are used for precise application to the lower and corner lashes.

8 Comb wands separate and define lashes.

9 Rubber brushes come in many shapes, and are generally better for separating and defining lashes.

10 Twisted wire brushes have irregularly spaced bristles, which have a more volumizing effect.

Anatomy of a mascara tube

The first mascara applicator tube was launched by Helena Rubinstein in 1957. The wiper insert is crucial for controlling the loading of the brush.

1. Straight brush

2. Curved brush

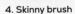

3. Hourglass brush

4. Skinny brush

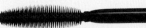

5. Tapered brush

6. Tapered brush

7. Ball tip brush

8. Comb wand

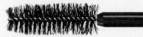

9. Rubber brush

10. Twisted wire

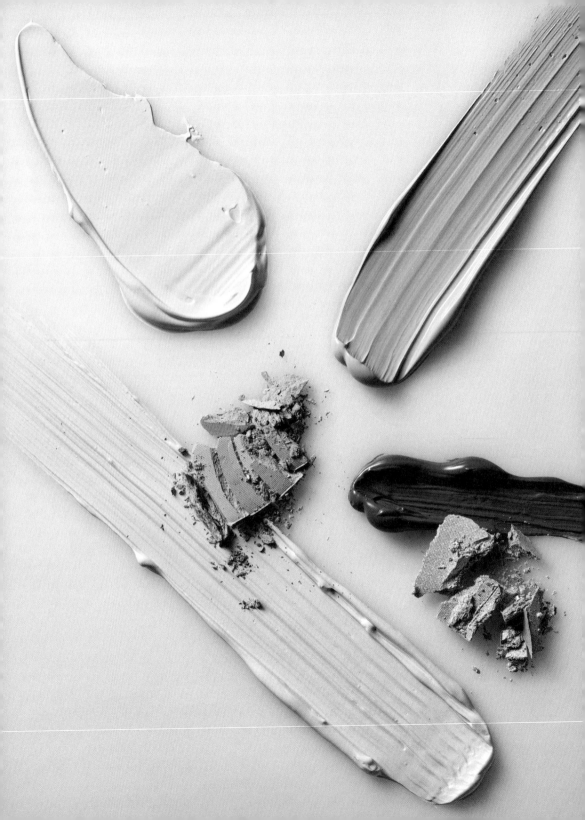

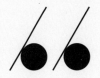

Lengthening mascaras
contain tiny nylon
or rayon fibres that
stick to the ends
of lashes.

What's in other eye makeup?

Eye makeup is an incredibly diverse category, with many different formulations and formats.

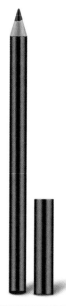

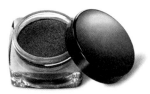

	CREAM AND LIQUID EYESHADOWS	PENCIL AND WIND-UP PRODUCTS
Formulation science	These usually contain pigments and powders suspended in an oily base. Some have an emulsion base, which feels lighter. Cream formulas are thickened with more waxes and clays than liquid formulas.	These are generally cream formulas, with added waxes to create a harder product. Eye products are formulated to apply smoothly, to avoid irritation. Pencils are made by injecting molten product into a wooden or plastic barrel. Poor formulas can partially absorb into the barrel, causing the remaining product to shrink and fall out. Cylinders for wind-up products are created by extrusion.
Tips	For longer-wearing, crease-resistant products, look for volatile solvents like isododecane, cyclopentasiloxane, or trisiloxane high on the ingredient list. These need to be blended with fingers or a brush before they set. Set these with a light veil of translucent powder – this also stops mascara from smearing on eyelids.	For intense colour and smoother application, warm pencils in your hands, or gently with a hair dryer (keep the lid on to prevent drying). Put pencils in the freezer before sharpening, to reduce crumbling. To avoid breaking wind-up products, only twist out a small amount at a time, and don't apply with too much force.

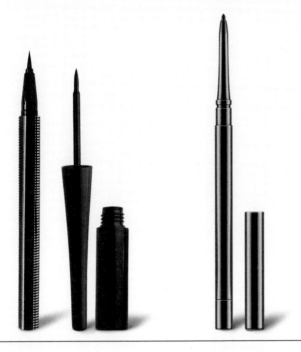

Here are some other routes to luscious lashes.

- **False eyelashes**
  These are glued to the skin above your lashes. Magnetic lashes stick to an iron-containing eyeliner or clamp onto the lashes.

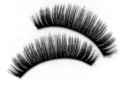

- **Eyelash extensions**
  Individual fibres are glued to each eyelash.

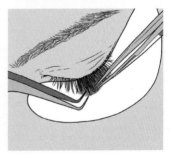

- **Lash tinting and lifting**
  Tinting uses oxidative dyes to colour the eyelashes, while lash lifts use perming products to reshape them. Both are risky as the alkaline products are corrosive to eyes.

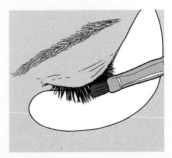

LIQUID EYELINER

Like mascaras (see pp192–193), these contain pigments in a volatile base, but have less waxes and powders so the dried film is thinner. Polymers add flexibility.

These usually come in tubes with a brush attached to the lid. Newer pens dispense the product from the barrel through a felt or brush tip.

Other products on the skin can collect on the applicator during use, and cause uneven lines. Remove build-up regularly by wiping the brush over a clean paper towel.

Felt-tip eyeliners can be easier to use, but they tend to be less pigmented since felt tips need thinner formulas.

GEL EYELINER

Pigments and polymers are suspended in a water-free base containing volatile solvents, which evaporate after application to leave a long-lasting film.

These originally came in pots and were applied with a separate brush, but gel products are increasingly found in speciality pencil and wind-up packaging, designed to prevent solvent escape.

Gel eyeliners can be blended like traditional pencils, but are far more transfer-resistant when set.

Close product lids tightly to stop solvents from evaporating.

Gel eyeliner brushes can be cleaned with two-phase makeup removers.

How do I remove makeup?

Regular cleansers can remove makeup, especially if it's light. But you can also use a dedicated makeup remover for heavier or water-resistant makeup.

Cleansers often sting eyes, so eye makeup removers are often preferred – these are designed to reduce irritation, such as with a slightly alkaline pH to match the eyes. To remove stubborn eye makeup, hold a pad soaked in remover over each eye for a few seconds to let makeup dissolve.

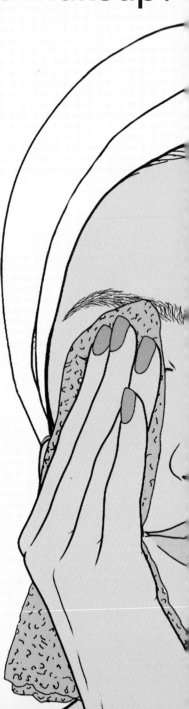

Cleansing oils and balms
Contain oils that can dissolve water-resistant makeup, along with surfactants which lift off the dirty oil. They are massaged on dry skin, then rinsed with water.

Makeup wipes
Usually contain solvents to dissolve makeup, before the wipe collects it. They are convenient, but overly enthusiastic wiping can be irritating and some wipes do not remove makeup very effectively. Many wipes are made of plastic fibres, and even biodegradable wipes can clog sewage systems if flushed.

Pure vegetable oils
These can be used to dissolve water-resistant makeup, but stay on skin unless removed with another cleanser.

Micellar waters
These no-rinse cleansers are dispensed onto cotton pads and wiped over skin. They usually contain mild surfactants that can be left on skin, but some formulas can be irritating if not rinsed off, particularly if skin is sensitive. They are a more sustainable alternative to makeup wipes, especially if used with reusable pads.

Cleansing creams and lotions ("cold creams")
Moisturizing emulsions that contain water to dissolve water-soluble dirt and sweat, and oil to dissolve water-resistant makeup. They are massaged into skin, then rinsed or wiped away.

Two-phase eye makeup removers
Contain a volatile oily layer and a water-based layer. They are shaken, dispensed onto a pad, then wiped over the eyes. These work as solvents, much like cleansing creams.

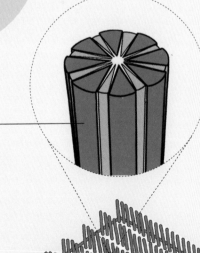

Split microfibre filament

Microfibre cloths
Sometimes marketed as "chemical-free" removers, these contain many tiny filaments bundled into strands that form a large surface area. When wetted and rubbed over skin, they collect makeup with friction on a tiny scale.

Do I need to wear sunscreen if my makeup has SPF?

SPF-rated makeup might make it seem like you can apply sunscreen and makeup in one time-saving step.

Unfortunately, it's unlikely that you'll apply enough of a makeup product to get adequate UV protection. You need to apply 2mg of product per square centimetre to achieve the labelled SPF, which translates to about a

quarter teaspoon (1.25g or $^1/_{20}$oz) of product on your face.

A very thick layer of an SPF-rated sheer foundation might give reasonable sun protection. But the vast majority of SPF-rated makeup products are designed primarily as makeup, to be used in far smaller quantities. To adequately protect your skin with makeup alone, you'd have to be absolutely caked in the stuff. At least SPF 30 is recommended when the UV index is 3 or higher. So while makeup

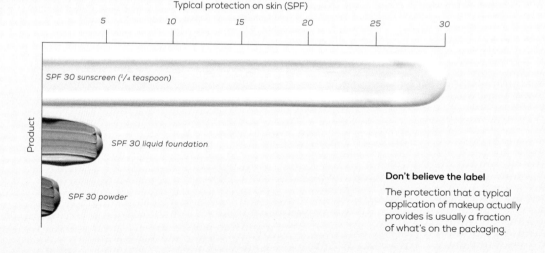

Typical protection on skin (SPF)

5   10   15   20   25   30

Product

SPF 30 sunscreen ($^1/_4$ teaspoon)

SPF 30 liquid foundation

SPF 30 powder

Don't believe the label

The protection that a typical application of makeup actually provides is usually a fraction of what's on the packaging.

Does it matter if I sleep in my makeup?

can contribute to sun protection, it isn't an adequate substitute for a dedicated sunscreen.

If you want to use a single product, tinted sunscreens are more likely to allow an effective application amount while doubling up as foundation. However, only limited shades are available, so finding a good colour match can be difficult. The most practical option for most people is to apply a generous layer of sunscreen or SPF moisturizer, then apply makeup gently on top.

A typical layer
of foundation containing
SPF 15 will equate to less
than SPF 1 on the skin
– effectively nothing.

Not removing your makeup can increase the chances of a breakout, but it's not inevitable.

In the past, it was thought that comedogenic ingredients would cause "acne cosmetica" – literally, breakouts caused by makeup. However, the evidence indicates that this varies from person to person, and product to product, even when worn overnight.

Some makeup contains irritating ingredients not found in skincare, like bismuth oxychloride. Makeup also collects pollutants and oxidized oils during the day, which can contribute to pore clogging and irritation – especially if left on the skin for a long time. Eye makeup can be extra risky (see pp210–211). Keep makeup wipes or micellar water next to your bed so you can remove your makeup even if you're exhausted.

What about "oil-free" makeup?

"Oil-free" products don't contain mineral or vegetable oils, which were mistakenly thought to cause acne in the past. However, whether makeup clogs your pores depends more on your skin chemistry and the overall formulation, rather than the presence or absence of specific ingredients.

How often do I need to clean my brushes?

Makeup brushes and tools can collect product residue, dead skin cells, and sebum, so they easily become contaminated with microbes, which are introduced to your face when you use them.

It's a good idea to clean your makeup brushes weekly to avoid irritation and breakouts, or more serious infections. Makeup tools should also be thoroughly disinfected before using them on a different person to avoid spreading infections.

To clean a brush quickly, spray the bristles with an alcohol-based brush cleaner and wipe on a paper towel.

Sponges can be cleaned by squeezing them in warm soapy water. You can also massage cleanser into them, then rinse by squeezing them under running water. If you don't have time to clean makeup tools, many products can be applied with your fingers or disposable tools.

HOW TO CLEAN YOUR BRUSHES

Brushes can be cleaned with shampoo, soap, or a brush-specific cleanser.

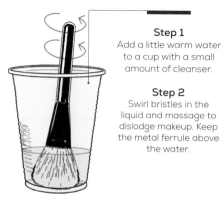

Step 1
Add a little warm water to a cup with a small amount of cleanser.

Step 2
Swirl bristles in the liquid and massage to dislodge makeup. Keep the metal ferrule above the water.

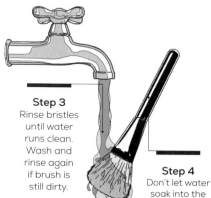

Step 3
Rinse bristles until water runs clean. Wash and rinse again if brush is still dirty.

Step 4
Don't let water soak into the handle – this can loosen the glue, warp the wood, and cause mould. Handles can be wiped clean with rubbing alcohol.

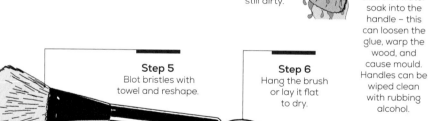

Step 5
Blot bristles with towel and reshape.

Step 6
Hang the brush or lay it flat to dry.

It's a good idea to clean your makeup brushes weekly to avoid irritation and breakouts, or more serious infections.

How does cosmetic tattooing work?

Cosmetic tattooing involves injecting pigment into the upper dermis with tiny needles. It is often used to mimic the look of makeup.

Unlike traditional tattoos, which are permanent, most modern cosmetic tattooing is semi-permanent, and meant to fade after a few years to allow for changing makeup trends. Ink tends to fade faster on oily skin, and with skincare products that increase skin turnover like exfoliants. Fading and colour changes can also occur with sun exposure. However, some of the injected pigment can last far longer, essentially becoming permanent. Pigment can also migrate and blur if placed too deep.

Eyebrow microblading is a form of semi-permanent makeup that uses a "blade" of needles to draw individual hair-like strokes. Other common cosmetic tattoos include eyeliner, lash enhancement (dots placed between lash hairs to make eyelashes look fuller), eyebrows, lips, and scalp micropigmentation.

Most cosmetic tattooing is performed with anaesthetic cream to minimize pain.

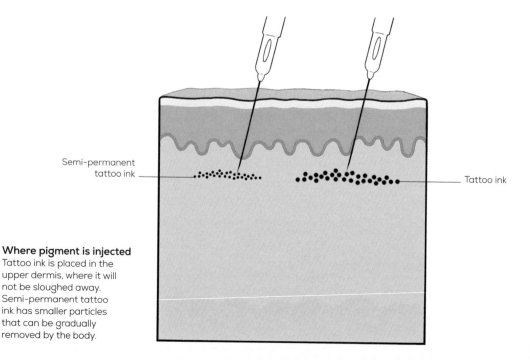

Semi-permanent tattoo ink

Tattoo ink

Where pigment is injected
Tattoo ink is placed in the upper dermis, where it will not be sloughed away. Semi-permanent tattoo ink has smaller particles that can be gradually removed by the body.

Risks

The risks of cosmetic tattooing are similar to other tattoos.

- Pigments can cause allergic and inflammatory reactions that lead to scarring, sometimes years after the initial procedure.
- Some pigment may be introduced deeper than intended, and become permanent. It can also change colour and blur. Complete pigment removal can be very difficult.

Proper aftercare is important for best results. Avoid wetting the tattooed area for around a week to support proper healing and minimize infection. Picking scabs can remove pigment and leave patchy areas.

Choosing a cosmetic tattooist

It's important to select a cosmetic tattooist carefully, as there is a high risk of infection and any mistakes can be permanently visible. Consider:

- What does their work look like, including after healing (e.g. six months later)? Is the colour natural and even? Does it match the style you want?
- How experienced is the tattooist, both at the type of tattooing you want and in general?

Ask for a consultation first so you can see what the clinic looks like, and do an allergy check. Infections are harmful to your health, and can ruin the results.

TATTOO HEALING PROCESS

After tattooing, it takes 4–6 weeks for skin to heal and the ink to settle.

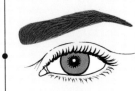

Day 1–2
Dark colour and some swelling may be present.

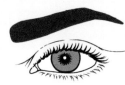

Day 3–5
Very dark colour, and scabbing may occur.

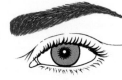

Day 6–9
Scabs fall off and colour appears patchy.

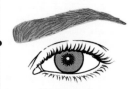

Day 10–14
The colour looks lighter.

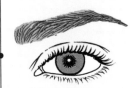

Day 14
From two weeks onwards the colour darkens to its final colour.

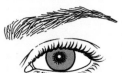

Day 42
After six weeks, the final results are achieved.

What order should I apply my makeup in?

You might have heard lots of conflicting advice about applying makeup, but the truth is, there are no strict rules!

Skincare generally goes under makeup. Start by cleansing the skin as usual and exfoliate if needed (see p70). Try to simplify your skincare products as they can cause makeup to shift more easily and crease faster. Remember to apply sunscreen (see pp84–85).

Applying makeup

Sunscreens sometimes have smoothing and illuminating effects and can work as primer.

Pore-filling primers contain silicone particles that can fill in pores and lines to create a smooth canvas.

Eyeshadow fallout is easier to clean up if applied before foundation.

Foundation is usually applied before concealer, as it provides some coverage, and can shift concealer if applied afterwards. A light layer of powder under foundation can help soak up excess oil.

SKINCARE ROUTINE

Prep your skin before applying makeup. You may not need all of these steps.

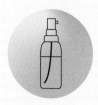

1. Cleanser
Removes dirt and oil.

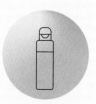

2. Toners or hydrating sprays
Lightweight products that tone and hydrate.

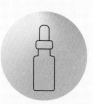

3. Serums and spot treatments
Products with concentrated skincare ingredients.

4. Moisturizer
Hydrates skin. May not be necessary if your other products are moisturizing enough.

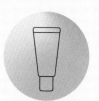

5. Sunscreen
Protects against daily UV damage.

Translucent powder can be used to set cream products before applying coloured powders to stop them from sticking unevenly.

Mascara should be applied after eyeshadow. Clamp-style lash curlers can remove mascara if used after application, sometimes taking lashes with it. Comb-style heated curlers can be used carefully after mascara. A fan can be used to set mascara faster, before lashes have a chance to drop.

Brow gel or pomade can help brow powder adhere, to create fuller brows.

Transparent lip liner or primer can fill in furrows and prevent feathering, without adding colour.

Makeup sprays can help with either finishing or fixing your makeup.

Pore-filling primers contain silicone particles that can fill in pores and lines to create a smooth canvas.

MAKEUP APPLICATION

These orders usually work well for the four main makeup categories. The categories themselves can be done in any order – some people prefer to apply complexion products before eye products, or vice versa. Use setting powder after cream and liquid products.

Complexion
1. Primer
2. Foundation
3. Concealer
4. Contour
5. Bronzer
6. Blush
7. Highlighter

Eyes
1. Primer
2. Cream or liquid eyeshadow
3. Powder eyeshadow
4. Eyeliner
5. Mascara

Brows
1. Powder
2. Pencil
3. Marker
4. Gel or pomade

Lips
1. Liner or primer
2. Lipstick
3. Lip gloss

How do I make my makeup last longer?

With longwear technologies in even the most budget-friendly makeup, it's easier than ever to make a full face of makeup last for hours. Here's how to make the most of these products.

Skin preparation

Sebum, sweat, and movement will eventually cause makeup to clump up and wear off. To help it last a full day, preparation is key:

- **Cleanse** Skin should be cleaned of any products or oils with a rinse-off cleanser, or by wiping with micellar water or toner.
- **Exfoliate** Dry skin flakes create crevices where makeup can gather over time. They can be removed with gentle physical exfoliation, like a damp cloth or peeling gel.
- **Moisturize** Hydrating skin makes it smoother, but only a small amount of moisturizer or primer should be used. Too much skincare can prevent makeup from forming an intact film and adhering to skin. Oily areas might not need a separate moisturizer, since makeup usually contains moisturizing ingredients. A mattifying primer can help absorb oil before it reaches the foundation film, but some silicone-rich primers can turn shiny after a few hours.

Dry skin should be thoroughly moisturized, otherwise makeup can settle into fine lines, look dull and cakey, and crack as the skin absorbs too much liquid from the makeup.

Combining products

Some skincare and makeup products can be incompatible and clump up quickly after application when used together. Make sure you test new combinations on your skin before use.

Tinted sunscreens and moisturizers can be a good way of reducing the number of products you're applying to your face, especially if you're only looking for light coverage. Many sunscreens can also have priming and moisturizing effects, so you may be able to skip a step.

Touch-ups

If your makeup needs to look good for hours, you will likely need to touch it up. Use moisturizing mists regularly to refresh makeup on dry skin. For oily skin, blot off oil before adding extra powder to reduce caking, and avoid high coverage powders.

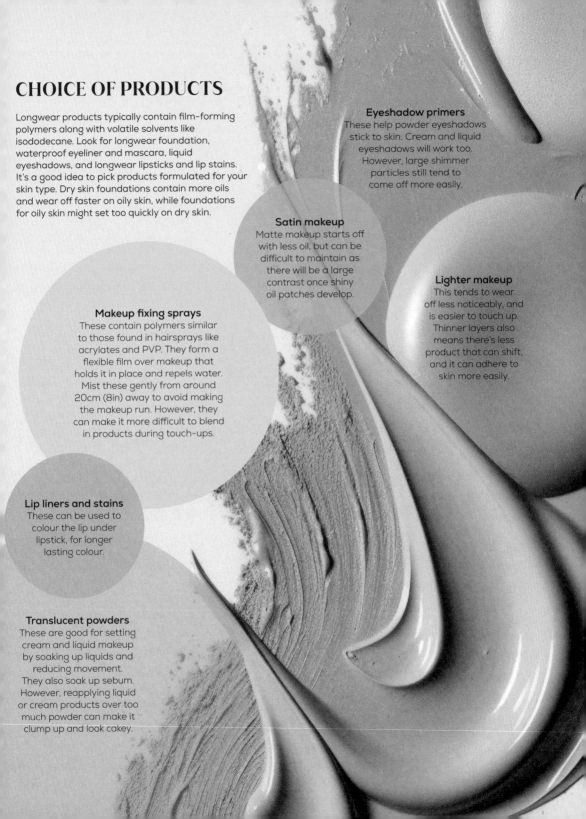

CHOICE OF PRODUCTS

Longwear products typically contain film-forming polymers along with volatile solvents like isododecane. Look for longwear foundation, waterproof eyeliner and mascara, liquid eyeshadows, and longwear lipsticks and lip stains. It's a good idea to pick products formulated for your skin type. Dry skin foundations contain more oils and wear off faster on oily skin, while foundations for oily skin might set too quickly on dry skin.

Eyeshadow primers

These help powder eyeshadows stick to skin. Cream and liquid eyeshadows will work too. However, large shimmer particles still tend to come off more easily.

Satin makeup

Matte makeup starts off with less oil, but can be difficult to maintain as there will be a large contrast once shiny oil patches develop.

Lighter makeup

This tends to wear off less noticeably, and is easier to touch up. Thinner layers also means there's less product that can shift, and it can adhere to skin more easily.

Makeup fixing sprays

These contain polymers similar to those found in hairsprays like acrylates and PVP. They form a flexible film over makeup that holds it in place and repels water. Mist these gently from around 20cm (8in) away to avoid making the makeup run. However, they can make it more difficult to blend in products during touch-ups.

Lip liners and stains

These can be used to colour the lip under lipstick, for longer lasting colour.

Translucent powders

These are good for setting cream and liquid makeup by soaking up liquids and reducing movement. They also soak up sebum. However, reapplying liquid or cream products over too much powder can make it clump up and look cakey.

Is eye makeup safe?

Your eyes are very sensitive organs that are prone to damage and infection, so there are heightened safety precautions for eye products.

For example, certain ingredients (including some pigments) are not approved for use in the eye area, and fragrance is usually omitted. Microbiological standards are also often stricter for eye products.

However, studies have still found potential risks. Makeup can migrate into the eye and scratch it, or interfere with structures that provide lubrication. Eye makeup users have a higher rate of eye dryness and irritation. In rare circumstances, pigment particles from mascara or eyeliner have become embedded into the surface of the eyeball or under the eyelid, with higher risk for contact lens wearers.

The biggest risk is still with infection, particularly with mascaras. Microbiological testing has found that microbes can build up within three months. Take note of when you started using a mascara, and discard it after three months. Do not thin mascaras with eye drops, water or saliva as this will likely compromise the preservative system.

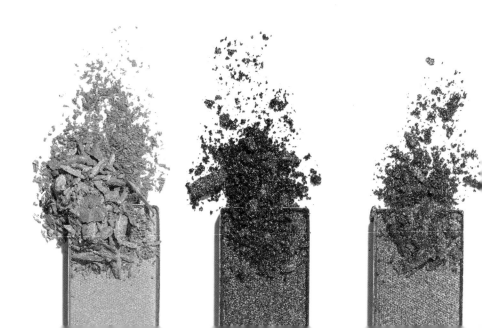

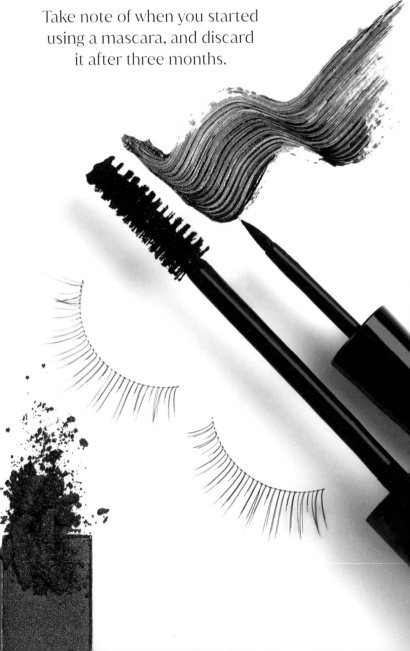

Take note of when you started using a mascara, and discard it after three months.

Using eye makeup safely
Follow these tips to protect your eyes.

- Only apply products designed for use near the eyes.

- Avoid eye makeup with large glittery particles, which can scratch the eyes.

- Don't share eye makeup with other people.

- Check the label (see p39) to see when you need to throw out your eye products.

- Remove false eyelashes very gently to avoid irritation or injury.

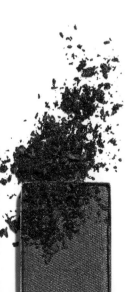

Are makeup ingredients dangerous?

Like other cosmetics, makeup products are assessed for safety, and ingredients are used at levels that are considered safe.

Pigments

Pigments are found in all colour cosmetics. Historically, many heavy metal compounds were used:
- Kohl eyeliner used by ancient Egyptians contained lead and copper.
- Red cinnabar blush used in ancient Rome and Elizabethan England contained mercury.

In most regions, pigments have special regulations, such as where they can be applied (e.g. not on lips) or permitted levels of contaminants. These regulations are based on toxicological assessments of risk (see pp12–15).

Common pigment concerns:
- "Coal tar colours" are the historical name for synthetic organic pigments (see pp180–181), due to how they were originally produced. They are highly purified, and cosmetic use has not been associated with any health concerns.
- Carbon black is essentially a purified form of soot. Health risks have been associated with contaminants in less purified versions not used in cosmetics.
- Titanium dioxide nanoparticles have been linked to cancer when inhaled. However, these are less white and are usually used as sunscreen filters, not pigments.
- Lead is a toxic heavy metal commonly found in the environment. It is naturally occurring, and was spread by the use of leaded petrol. Lead can sometimes contaminate makeup products, and is of particular concern for lip products since they can be swallowed. Levels in lip products are limited to below 0.001% in most countries, and the concentrations measured in commercially available lipsticks are almost always well below this limit.
- Traditional eye cosmetics containing kohl or kajal often contain high levels of lead, even if labelled "lead-free". These can cause neurological problems, particularly in children. Other toxic heavy metals like arsenic and cadmium have also been detected. These products are illegal in many countries, but easily purchased online.

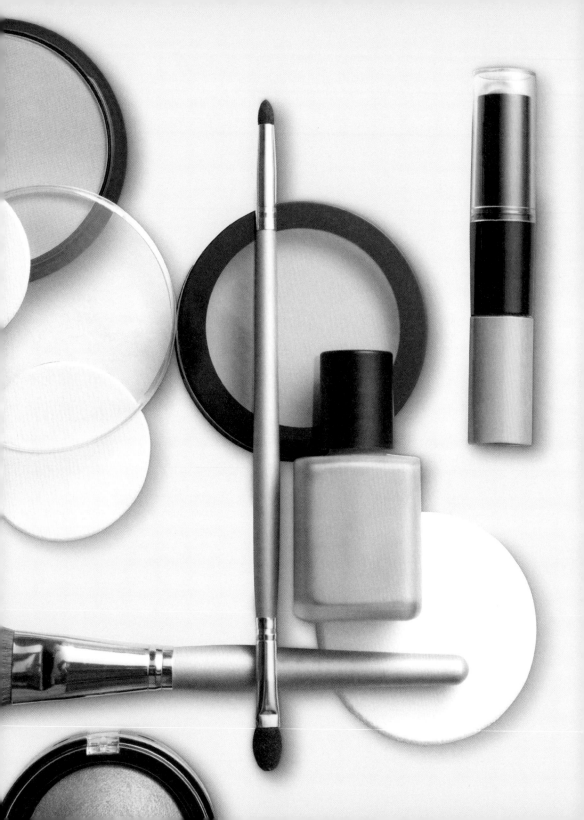

Levels of lead in lip products are limited to below 0.001%, and the concentrations measured in commercially available lipsticks are usually well below this limit.

Silicones

Silicones are used in many makeup products to help them spread smoothly and form durable films. There are myths about silicones suffocating skin and clogging pores, but the evidence does not support these claims. The environmental hazards of cyclotetrasiloxane and cyclopentasiloxane have led to reductions in the allowed levels in some products, although there is disagreement amongst experts about the actual risk.

Per- and polyfluoroalkyl substances (PFAS)

PFAS are substances with high fluorine content. They are commonly used in water-repellent fabrics, non-stick cookware, and fire-fighting foams, but they do not break down easily and have become persistent environmental pollutants. Some PFAS have been linked to high cholesterol, lowered immune responses, and cancer.

In cosmetics, some PFAS are used in waterproof makeup products at very low concentrations (usually well under 0.1%) or as impurities. However, they are uncommon (intentionally used by less than 1.5% of companies in a 2020 survey) and use is further declining as their risks have become better known. They generally do not penetrate skin easily, so the highest risk

is likely with water-resistant lip products. Exposure from cosmetics would be very low compared to dietary intake.

Talc and asbestos

Talc is a naturally occurring mineral used in many makeup products, as well as talcum powders. Deposits of talc are sometimes found near asbestos, a spiky mineral widely used in buildings before the 1980s that can cause cancer (mesothelioma) if inhaled. Cosmetic talc is required to be asbestos-free, but traces of asbestos have been found in a few eyeshadows and baby powders.

However, these appear to be isolated cases of contamination. Between 2019 and 2022, the FDA tested 152 talc-containing products from 90 different brands, and found asbestos in products from 3 brands only. Higher mesothelioma rates have not been recorded in demographics who use a lot of makeup or baby powder.

Exposure to talc from makeup is low, given the small amounts used. The potential link between the use of powder in the genital area and ovarian cancer has also been investigated since the 1960s. In 2020 an analysis of pooled data from a quarter million women found no association, although a small increase in risk could not be ruled out.

How can I look more awake?

Makeup can transform your appearance, which comes in handy for hiding a bad night's sleep.

Makeup can be used to emphasize particular features and downplay others. Highlighting products can bring forward areas of skin, while contouring products create the illusion of shadow.

Larger eyes

Larger-looking eyes can make you appear more awake. Studies have found that eyeliner and mascara can make eyes appear larger. This is similar to the Delboeuf illusion, where a border closely surrounding an object makes it look bigger. Experiment with different eyeliner thicknesses and techniques to see what best compliments your eye shape. Grey or navy eyeliner can make the whites of eyes look brighter, and define eyes more subtly. Curl your lashes before applying mascara to maximize the effect.

Use a white or beige pencil to line the lower waterline to widen eyes and disguise redness. Open up the eyes with a little light eyeshadow or highlighter near the inner and outer corners.

False eyelashes with the longest part of the lash in the centre makes eyes look more open.

EYELINER AND EYE SIZE

In an experiment, different levels of eyeliner made the eye look different sizes (% by area). Not lining the entire eye allows colour assimilation, where light areas of skin are perceived to add to the eye area.

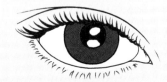

No eyeliner
The eye with no makeup was used as a reference (area of 100%).

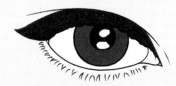

Upper eyeliner
Wearing eyeliner on the upper lid increased the perceived size to 109%.

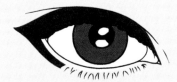

Upper and lower
Adding eyeliner to one third of the lower lid increased the perceived size to 111%, but fully lining the lower lid reduced this to 107%.

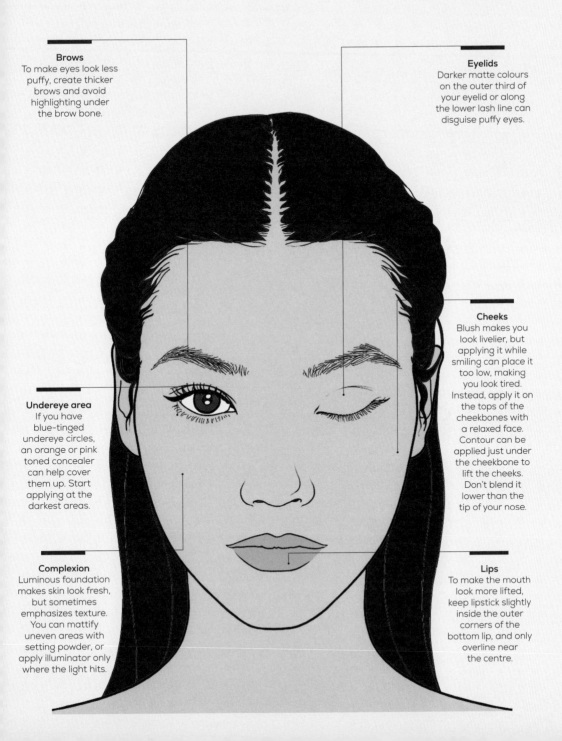

Brows
To make eyes look less puffy, create thicker brows and avoid highlighting under the brow bone.

Eyelids
Darker matte colours on the outer third of your eyelid or along the lower lash line can disguise puffy eyes.

Cheeks
Blush makes you look livelier, but applying it while smiling can place it too low, making you look tired. Instead, apply it on the tops of the cheekbones with a relaxed face. Contour can be applied just under the cheekbone to lift the cheeks. Don't blend it lower than the tip of your nose.

Undereye area
If you have blue-tinged undereye circles, an orange or pink toned concealer can help cover them up. Start applying at the darkest areas.

Complexion
Luminous foundation makes skin look fresh, but sometimes emphasizes texture. You can mattify uneven areas with setting powder, or apply illuminator only where the light hits.

Lips
To make the mouth look more lifted, keep lipstick slightly inside the outer corners of the bottom lip, and only overline near the centre.

Nails

What are nails made of?

Our nails protect our fingers, improve our sense of touch, and help us pick up small objects. Like hair, they are rich in keratin proteins that are responsible for many of their properties, including their unusual strength.

Nail matrix

The matrix sits under the skin near the knuckle. Matrix cells divide to produce nail cells (onychocytes), which flatten, die, and harden to form the nail plate. Part of the matrix can sometimes be seen as the white lunula.

Nail plate

Fingernails grow around 3mm ($^1/_8$in) a month. The nail plate slides along the nail bed as it grows, and separates at the fingertip to form the free edge, which appears white. The flat, tile-like nail cells contain tough keratin proteins. Like in hair, many bonds crosslink adjacent protein strands to make nails harder.

The surface layer of the nail is the dorsal layer. It is hard, with many crosslinked proteins. Beneath this is the thick intermediate layer, which contains strong keratin fibres lying across the width of the nail. This is why nails tend to break sideways, instead of deeper into the living nail bed – it takes twice the energy to

CROSS-SECTION OF A NAIL

Here we take a microscopic view of the nail layers, which all play a part in creating strength and resilience.

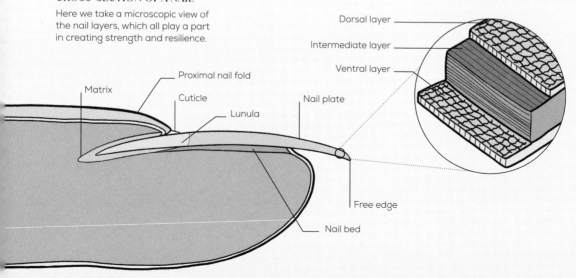

Dorsal layer

Intermediate layer

Ventral layer

Proximal nail fold

Matrix

Cuticle

Lunula

Nail plate

Free edge

Nail bed

cut a nail along its length. The final layer is the ventral layer, which is attached to the nail bed.

Nail bed and skin

Nail beds have epidermal and dermal layers like the rest of our skin. Ridges run along the direction of growth, which match the ridges on the underside of the nail. Blood vessels in the dermis can be seen as a pink colour through each nail. The nail plate is quite permeable to water but not much else – water from the nail bed evaporates through the nail.

Nail folds seal the nail plate along three sides, protecting the living tissue from infection. The proximal nail fold sits over the matrix. It is often mistakenly called the cuticle, which is actually the thin film of dead cells that travels on the nail's surface as it grows. The onychodermal band sits under the nail before the free edge, and seals the final side.

Why do nails break?

Like with hair, nail properties change a lot with hydration. Water breaks crosslinking hydrogen bonds between proteins, so too much water makes the nails weak and overly flexible, while too little water makes the nails brittle, so they crack with impact instead of bending. 18% water content is ideal.

The geometry of the nail also contributes to its strength. Curves both across and along the nail spread forces more evenly. Flatter nails bend and break more easily.

NAIL OIL

Nails naturally contain a small amount of oil which adds flexibility. This can be supplemented with nail oils.

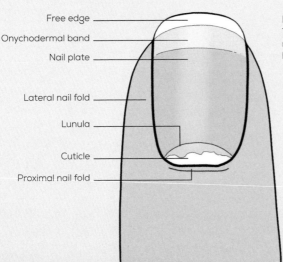

Free edge
Onychodermal band
Nail plate
Lateral nail fold
Lunula
Cuticle
Proximal nail fold

Parts of the nail

The skin around and under the nail can be as important to nail health as the nail plate itself.

How do I look after my nails?

Even if you aren't concerned about how your nails look, it's still important to maintain them to avoid pain and infection.

Cutting and filing nails

It's best to cut nails when they're hydrated, like after a shower, as they are more flexible and any cracks will travel less. However, you should file nails when they're dry, using a fine-to-medium grit file to reduce splitting and peeling. Any jagged edges that might catch on fabrics should be filed smooth.

Some nail shapes are more hard-wearing. Short oval nails that follow the shape of each fingertip are least prone to breakage. Sections of the free edge further from the fingertip break more easily since they are less supported, like the corners of square nails. They also tend to be more brittle as there is less hydration from the underlying skin.

Buffing nails

Most people have ridges running along the surface of their nails. You can smooth these down very conservatively with a buffing file, but this will thin and weaken the nail, and should be avoided if your nails are already fragile.

Cuticle removal

The nail folds form a seal against microbes. During manicures, the proximal nail fold (often mistakenly called "the cuticle", see

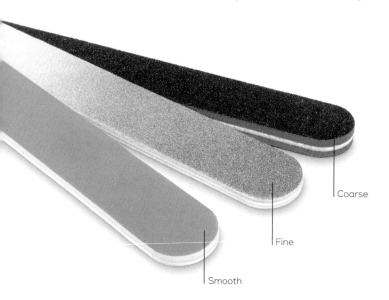

Coarse

Fine

Smooth

Choosing a nail file
Nail files come in different textures. "Grit" refers to the number of surface grains that fit into a square inch. Smoother files with higher grit numbers are less likely to damage nails.

p221) is sometimes aggressively pushed back or cut, which risks infection. In some cases, the nail matrix can be damaged which permanently affects nail growth.

Liquid cuticle removers are a safer option. These contain sodium or potassium hydroxide (<5%) which breaks up cuticle remnants and excess dead skin. Acid exfoliants can also slough off dead skin. Regular use can keep the skin around the nails neat and prevent hangnails. However, cuticle removers are caustic, so make sure you follow the instructions. The edge of the proximal nail fold should only be pushed back very gently, after soaking in water to soften.

Buffing will thin and weaken the nail, and should be avoided if your nails are already fragile.

NAIL SHAPE

Here are some popular nail shapes. Filing before removing nail polish can make it easier to see the nail shape and keep it symmetrical.

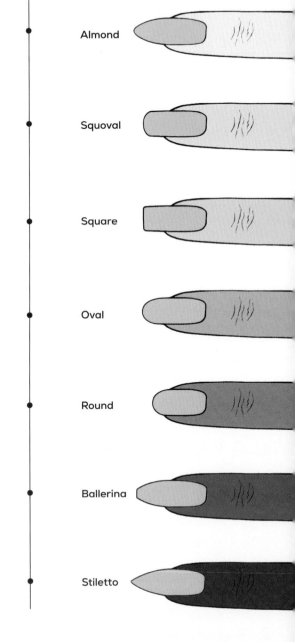

Almond

Squoval

Square

Oval

Round

Ballerina

Stiletto

What's in nail polish?

Modern nitrocellulose-based nail polishes were developed in the 1920s, inspired by new paints developed for cars.

After application, solvents evaporate to leave a tough, waterproof film that's stuck firmly to the nail, and lasts for up to a week.

Main components

Colouring agents in nail polish are usually brightly coloured organic lake pigments (see pp180–181). Pearlescent and metallic pigments are added for shimmer or glitter finishes.

Polymers are long molecules that make up most of the nail polish film. Multiple polymers are used to adjust the adhesion, hardness, and glossiness.

Plasticizers keep the film flexible to prevent chipping when the nail bends. They sit between polymer chains, preventing them from sticking together too tightly.

Solvents dissolve ingredients, and control texture and drying time. They evaporate quickly to minimize smudging and dents, but if the polish dries too fast it can chip easily and trap bubbles. Organic solvents like ethyl acetate, butyl acetate, and isopropyl alcohol are used. These are resistant to microbial growth, so additional preservatives are not needed.

Viscosity modifiers keep pigments suspended and adjust the texture.

UV filters protect the polish colour from changing with UV exposure.

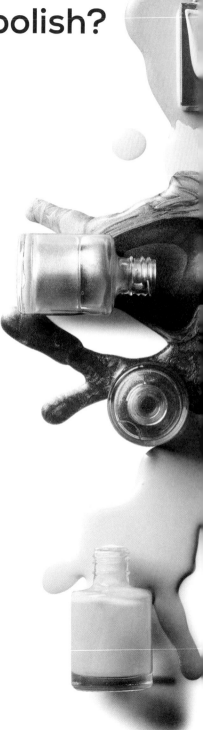

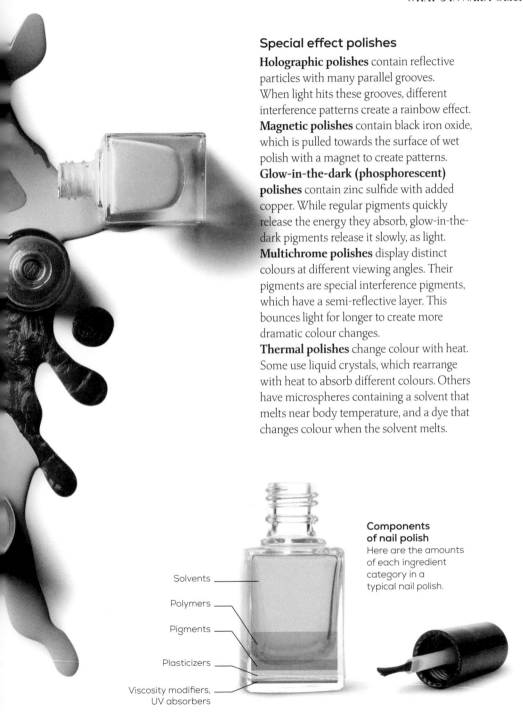

Special effect polishes

Holographic polishes contain reflective particles with many parallel grooves. When light hits these grooves, different interference patterns create a rainbow effect.

Magnetic polishes contain black iron oxide, which is pulled towards the surface of wet polish with a magnet to create patterns.

Glow-in-the-dark (phosphorescent) polishes contain zinc sulfide with added copper. While regular pigments quickly release the energy they absorb, glow-in-the-dark pigments release it slowly, as light.

Multichrome polishes display distinct colours at different viewing angles. Their pigments are special interference pigments, which have a semi-reflective layer. This bounces light for longer to create more dramatic colour changes.

Thermal polishes change colour with heat. Some use liquid crystals, which rearrange with heat to absorb different colours. Others have microspheres containing a solvent that melts near body temperature, and a dye that changes colour when the solvent melts.

Components of nail polish

Here are the amounts of each ingredient category in a typical nail polish.

Solvents

Polymers

Pigments

Plasticizers

Viscosity modifiers, UV absorbers

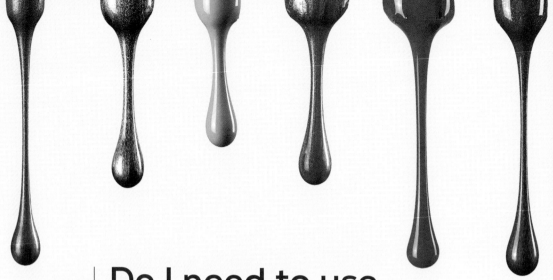

Do I need to use "10-free" nail polish?

Nail polishes often market themselves as being "free from" a number of ingredients. This number has grown over the years, and has largely become a marketing competition between brands.

"10-free" nail polishes are formulated without ten ingredients that have been deemed to be potentially harmful. However, as the nail plate is quite impervious to most substances, avoiding skin contact with polish and applying in a well-ventilated area will reduce any exposures immensely.

3-Free

"Free" labels started with "3-free". The vast majority of nail polishes have been 3-free for a few decades, meaning they do not contain:

Dibutyl phthalate (DBP) A plasticizer, linked to endocrine effects. The amounts in polish were not expected to have any health impacts, and were extremely low compared to other sources like food. It was banned in 2007 as a precaution in EU cosmetics, and most brands phased it out soon after.

Toluene A solvent that causes birth defects, nausea, and organ damage with prolonged recreational use. The amounts in nail polish are too low to have these effects.

Formaldehyde Nail hardeners contain methylene glycol or formalin, which release formaldehyde in small amounts to crosslink nail proteins. It can cause nasal cancers if inhaled in large quantities, but the amounts from nail products are low, with the concentrations measured in nail salons similar to those in homes. However, it can cause allergies and irritation, and can make nails brittle if overused.

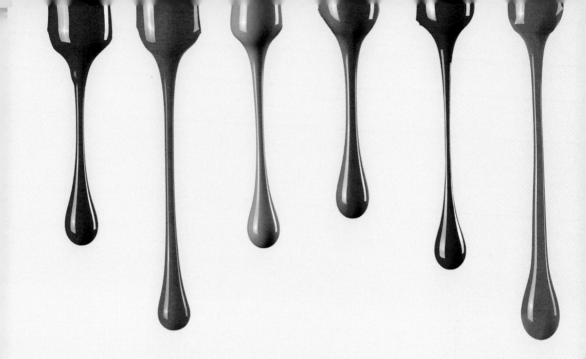

4-Free

Additionally, "4-free" polishes do not contain:

Tosylamide/formaldehyde resin
Improves adhesion to the nail. This sometimes contains very low (0.5%) levels of formaldehyde as an impurity, which can be an issue for people with allergies.

5-Free

"5-free" polishes also do not contain:

Camphor A naturally occurring plasticizer that can irritate skin, but not at the low concentrations used in nail polish. It's found in far higher amounts in herbs like rosemary.

OTHER INGREDIENTS IN "FREE FROM" LISTS

Ethyl tosylamide
A plasticizer. In some regions, it seems to have been mistakenly banned by overly broad regulations, as it has structural similarities to sulfa antibiotics. It may irritate skin, but this is unlikely at the amounts used in nail polish.

Triphenyl phosphate (TPHP)
A plasticizer, also used as a flame retardant in other applications. A study detected increased amounts in urine after nail polish use, but these levels were still very low.

Gluten, fragrance, acetone
Only a concern for people with allergies to those ingredients.

Parabens, xylene, sulfates, lead, methylisothiazolinone, bisphenol A, nonylphenol ethoxylates, styrene, 4-methoxyphenol (MEHQ), tert-butyl hydroperoxide
Never used or extremely rare in nail polish, for at least the last few decades.

How do I make nail polish last longer?

Here are some tips to help you apply nail polish more smoothly and make your manicure last.

Preparation

Apply nail polish to dry nails. Nails change shape as they dry, which can lead to lifting. Don't over-buff the nail as it can make it thin and flexible, leading to poor adhesion.

Remove the dead cuticle on the nail (see pp222–223) as it can block polish from bonding to the nail, leading to lifting.

Mix the nail polish by rolling the bottle. Shaking can create bubbles. Check the texture of the nail polish as solvents can evaporate over time. Thickened polishes trap more bubbles and stop brush marks from flattening out. Add nail polish thinner until the polish is the right consistency. Do not add nail polish remover as it contains ingredients that can drastically change the formula, like acetone or water.

Application

Wipe the nail surface with nail polish remover immediately before application. This removes any oily residues or old polish, so the polish can bind more effectively.

Apply a base coat. These contain polymers that stick better to the nail, reducing chipping and wear. They also act as a barrier to prevent pigment stains.

Special base coats can strengthen nails or fill in ridges. Extend the base coat, polish, and top coat over the tip of the nail to reduce wear.

Apply two or three thin layers of polish to give a uniform colour. Thick layers can shrink and wrinkle as they dry, and chip more easily. Let the polish dry slowly, without blowing, to reduce shrinkage and give a smoother, shinier finish. Letting each layer dry slightly before applying the next can also help.

Apply a top coat to help the manicure last. These contain more hard and glossy polymers, plus UV filters to give additional colour protection. Cellulose acetate butyrate is often the main polymer as it does not turn yellow in light as quickly as nitrocellulose.

A UV-cured gel top coat can be used on completely dry nail polish for even more durability (see pp230–231).

Maintenance

Avoid excessive sun exposure. UV can discolour nail polish and make it brittle.

Minimize contact with water, which makes nails flex and detaches the polish. Wear gloves when washing dishes or cleaning. This also reduces exposure to cleaning agents that can break down the polish.

Avoid mechanical wear like scratching and rubbing as much as possible.

How do I remove nail polish?

Nail polish removers contain solvents that redissolve the polish film by breaking temporary bonds between polymer molecules.

Acetone is one of the most effective solvents for removing nail polish, and is very safe. Alternatives like ethyl acetate or methyl diesters usually work less effectively and are not necessarily safer. Solvents also remove water and oil from the nail and surrounding skin. Look for glycerin and oils in removers to counteract any drying, and moisturize your hands and nails afterwards.

Technique

Soak cotton wool or tissue in remover and wipe it over each nail. For more stubborn polishes like glitters, you can place a remover-soaked pad on each nail and wrap your fingertips in foil. After 5–10 minutes, the polish should slide off easily. You can file off the top layers before removal so solvent can soak in more easily. Nail polish removers should be used in a well-ventilated area, as the smells can cause headaches. Never peel off nail polish as the surface layers of the nail can come off with it.

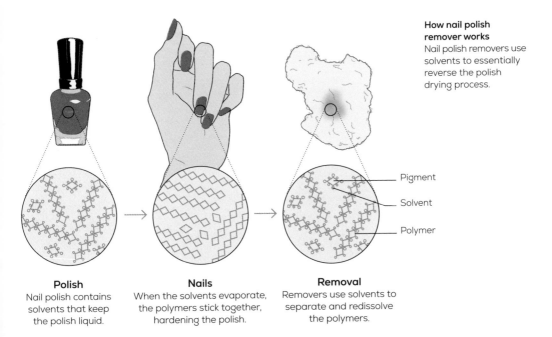

How nail polish remover works
Nail polish removers use solvents to essentially reverse the polish drying process.

Pigment

Solvent

Polymer

Polish
Nail polish contains solvents that keep the polish liquid.

Nails
When the solvents evaporate, the polymers stick together, hardening the polish.

Removal
Removers use solvents to separate and redissolve the polymers.

How do acrylics, gels, and dip powders work?

Traditional nail polish typically only lasts for around a week before chipping. For harder-wearing nails, a whole different chemical process is needed.

The key components in nail products are polymers, which are long chains made of many joined-up monomers. But while nail polish already contains the final polymers, longer-lasting products like acrylics, gels, and dip powders join up their monomers after application, in a process called polymerization or "curing".

Some products include crosslinking monomers, which add reinforcing bonds between polymer chains. More crosslinks result in a more durable and rigid final material, which can be used for sculptured nail extensions.

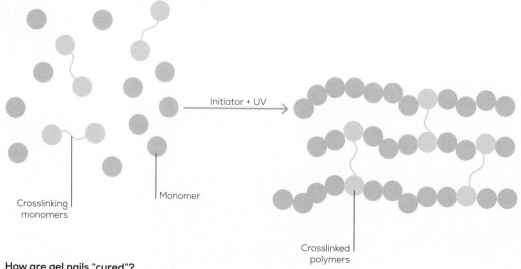

Initiator + UV

Crosslinking monomers

Monomer

Crosslinked polymers

How are gel nails "cured"?
Durable nail products like gels contain monomers, which join up on the nail to create tough polymer networks. Crosslinks provide additional strength.

Acrylic nails

Acrylic nail products were originally inspired by dental resins. They consist of a powder and a liquid that are mixed just before application. The powder is made up of polymer beads and an initiator, which starts the polymerization reaction. The liquid contains monomers and a catalyst to activate the initiator.

During application, the liquid and powder are mixed, then dabbed onto the nail. The catalyst and initiator start a chain reaction that joins up the monomers into a polymer network around the powder beads. The acrylic is hard after a few minutes, although complete polymerization takes a few days.

	NAIL POLISH	ACRYLIC	GEL	DIP POWDER
Monomers	None	Ethyl methacrylate	Methacrylates (e.g. HEMA)	Cyanoacrylates
Pre-formed polymers	Nitrocellulose and other polymers	Solid polymethacrylate beads	Liquid oligomers (small polymers)	Solid polymethacrylate beads
Polymerization initiated by	None	Initiator (benzoyl peroxide) reacts with catalyst (dimethyltolylamine)	Initiator (e.g. a phenylphosphinate) reacts upon UV exposure	Water
Other product features		Inhibitor (hydroquinone) prevents monomers from curing too early	Light protective packaging prevents early polymerization	Accelerator contains an alkaline catalyst dimethyltolylamine to speed up polymerization
Uses	Overlays	Overlays Nail tips Sculptured extensions	Overlays Nail tips Sculptured extensions (hard gel or builder-in-a-bottle)	Overlays Nail tips
Lasts for	Up to a week	2–3 weeks	2–3 weeks	2–3 weeks

Gel nails

Gel products use UV instead of a catalyst to activate the initiator and join up monomers, so all their components are in the one product. Like acrylics they contain liquid monomers, but instead of solid polymer beads they use small liquid polymers (oligomers) to avoid blocking UV. There is also a UV-activated initiator to start polymerization.

Traditional gels were thick and difficult to apply. Newer gel polish and "builder-in-a-bottle" products that apply like nail polish have made gels far more popular.

Special longer-lasting nail polishes incorporate gel-like technology, but their components join up with natural light exposure, without a UV lamp. They last for up to two weeks.

Dip powders

Dip powder manicures involve applying a monomer liquid to the nail, followed by coloured polymer powder. Water causes the monomers to join up. Liquid and powder layers are repeated to build up the coating.

Similarities and differences

While these nail products are similar, there are some differences that can make one a better choice for your needs.

Acrylic tends to be more hard-wearing, while gel is more resistant to cleaning chemicals. Dip powders are easier to apply and produce less odours. All three use monomers, which can cause allergies. This risk depends on the skill of the nail technician:

- Allergy risk increases if monomers touch the skin.
- Since acrylic products require mixing, using the wrong ratio of monomer to initiator can make a weak acrylic that cracks or lifts, or leave unreacted monomer, which can cause allergies.
- For gel the ratio is predetermined, but incorrect curing can cause similar problems. A mismatched lamp can deliver the wrong dose of UV. If the UV is too intense, heat can be produced very quickly during polymerization and cause burns. Insufficient UV leaves unreacted monomers, which can cause allergies – for example, using an old or dirty lamp, or if too thick a layer is applied and UV can't reach the bottom.
- Dip liquids can cause respiratory allergies that results in flu-like symptoms, if ventilation is insufficient.

All three products are removed by soaking in acetone to loosen the polymer network, then gently pushing off the nail. Hard gels need to be filed off.

What does a salon manicure involve?

Salons provide different services to maintain and enhance your nails.

A standard manicure involves shaping your nails and applying nail polish. The skin around your nails might also be tidied, or you may receive a hand massage.

More durable nail products, such as acrylic, gel, and dip systems (see previous pages) can be used for longer-lasting treatments.

> Acrylic, gel, and dip manicures last for 2–3 weeks.

OVERLAYS AND EXTENSIONS

Acrylic, gel, and dip manicures last for 2–3 weeks. These are some of the ways they can be used.

Overlay
Overlays are thin films applied on the natural nail, like nail polish.

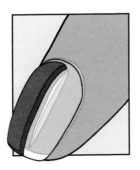

Sculptured extensions
Sculptured nail extensions are more durable than tips. A paper template (form) is stuck under the nail edge to act as a base, then product is applied with a brush and cured.

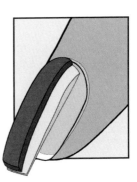

Nail tips
Nail tips made of plastic can be glued to the free edge. These are filed to the desired shape, then an overlay is added to reinforce the connection.

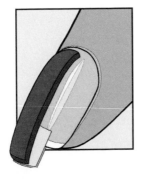

Infill
As the nail grows, extra product can be added to cover up the bare nail (infill) or the artificial nail may be thinned and product reapplied to adjust the shape (rebalance).

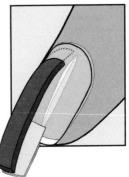

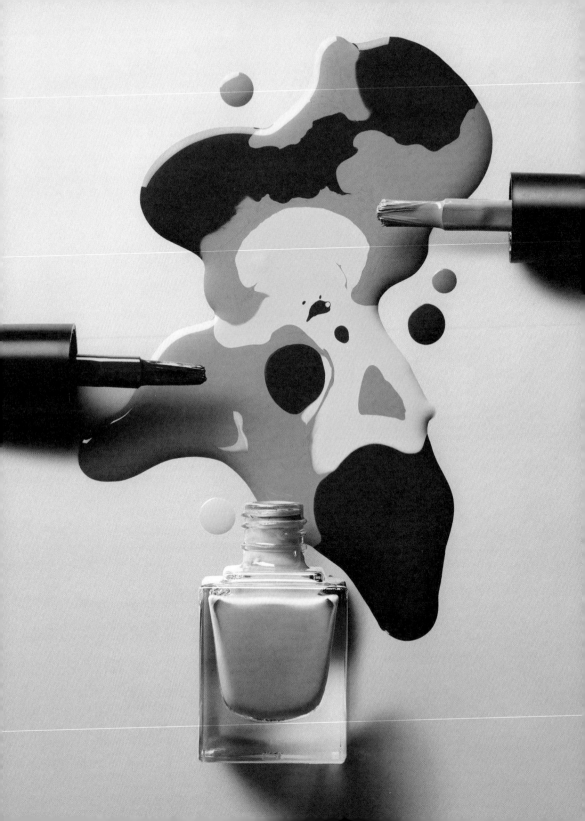

As the nail plate is quite
impervious to most
substances, avoiding
skin contact with polish
and applying in a well-
ventilated area will
reduce any exposures.

Are manicures bad for me?

Nail services come with risks, but they can be reduced by experienced nail technicians.

Nail damage

Nail polish, overlays, and extensions can make your nails better or worse. They can reinforce and protect thin nails as they grow, and create a barrier that keeps the water content of nails more consistent. However, nail polish remover can strip away oil and water, and improper product application and removal can cause damage.

Here are some further points to consider when applying and removing nail products.

Nail separation
Long rigid extensions can act as levers and cause nail separation, especially if the nails are used as tools.

Heat spikes
Gel polymerization produces heat. If the lamp is too strong, monomers react too quickly, causing a painful heat spike. In extreme cases, the nail can separate from the nail bed.

Excessive filing
Filing the nail surface helps polymerizable products adhere. However, excessive filing thins the nails, making them weaker and more sensitive to allergens and heat.

APPLICATION

MMA
Acrylics that use methyl methacrylate (MMA) are more rigid and can cause nail separation. MMA has been largely phased out or banned, but can still be found in grey market products.

Poor technique
Nails can separate with improperly applied products, like thick gel layers that shrink when cured.

Soak-off products

Soak your nails until the product (e.g. gel) is loose enough to come off easily. Forcing it off can cause severe pitting on the nail, which is especially fragile after soaking.

Careful filing

Removing nail products often involves filing, which can cause damage if not done carefully.

REMOVAL

Nourishing ingredients

Look for removers containing humectants like glycerin, and use oils and moisturizers after removal.

Increased fragility

Even without damage, nails can feel weak for about a day after removal due to increased hydration. Be careful with your nails until they regain their rigidity.

CHOOSING A SAFE NAIL SALON

Before trying a new nail salon, make a note of the following:

- **Hygiene and cleanliness**
Observe and ask about their hygiene procedures. Is the salon clean and free of spills? Are stations cleaned between clients? Is food eaten at stations? Do technicians wear gloves and change them regularly? Are tools disinfected between clients? Are containers closed after use? Is there double-dipping with products?

- **Staff safety**
Is the salon well-ventilated, or do odours linger? While risks should be low for customers even with poor ventilation, a salon that cuts corners when looking after their staff are more likely to do the same elsewhere. Are employees appropriately qualified? Check that any regulations for nail salons in your area are followed.

Infection

Infections can occur in salons where proper hygiene procedures aren't followed (see previous page). Improperly cleaned tools and equipment like foot spas can spread infections.

Manicures should be performed gently – microbes collect under the nail, so aggressive filing and cleaning can break the skin and introduce microbes into the living tissue. Rough treatment of the nail folds can also cause infection.

Nails should be disinfected before applying longwear nail products, as trapped microbes can cause an infection. If the product cracks, repair or remove it quickly, as microbes can enter and grow.

Allergies

Allergies to nail product monomers have been increasing, especially with the rise of home gel kits. These cause itching and redness, misshapen nails, and nail separation. Smaller monomers that were more likely to cause allergic reactions have been replaced in many products. Other ingredients like UV filters and initiators can also cause allergies. Allergy risk increases with exposure so avoid the following:

• Skin contact when excess product spills over from the nail.
• Touching the "sticky" layer on top of cured product.
• Inhaling or touching filing dust.
• Incomplete curing, as monomers can absorb through the nail (see p232).
• Applying products to damaged or overly thin nails.

Chemical exposure

Nail salons use substances that can potentially build up to harmful levels with inadequate ventilation. This is not a substantial risk for customers who go there for a few hours a week, but can be dangerous for workers who are exposed continuously. Ingredients with strong odours can cause headaches and nausea even at safe levels. Inhaled dusts can be irritating and contribute to allergies.

BEAUTY MYTHS

NAILS NEED TO "BREATHE"

It's a myth that nails need to "breathe" or rest between nail products. Nail cells are dead, and the nail bed receives nutrients from blood vessels. Frequent removal is more likely to damage the nail plate than the products themselves.

Are nail lamps dangerous?

Nail lamps for curing gel products use mostly long wavelengths of UVA over 350 nm, which can increase the risk of skin cancers and premature skin aging.

Lamps produce different amounts and wavelengths of UVA and UVB, and there is some uncertainty about the impacts of repeated exposure to narrow bands of UVA. Lamps in home kits are also not well regulated.

There have been a few reports of people developing skin cancers on their hands after many years of regular gel manicures. However, it is unclear whether they were the cause, as these cases usually involved other predisposing factors like tanning bed use or photosensitizing medications. It's possible that in rare cases, nail lamps could increase skin cancer risk in susceptible people.

Nail lamp emissions

Multiple studies have measured the amounts of UV received during a typical gel manicure. UVB exposure is negligible (equivalent to 6–10 minutes exposure below UV index 2), while UVA is moderate (similar to 6–10 minutes of midday sun in summer in Barcelona).

Some simple steps can drastically reduce any risk:

- **Apply a broad spectrum sunscreen** to your hands before gel manicures. Wipe nails with remover afterwards to ensure good adhesion.
- **Wear UV protective gloves** that only expose the fingertips during gel manicures.
- **Avoid looking at UV lights.**
- **Don't get gel manicures** when taking medications that increase light sensitivity, or if you have a photosensitizing condition.
- **Don't use UV lamps** to dry products that don't need UV.
- **Use UV-free products** if you plan to change your nails frequently.
- **Monitor your hands** for any suspicious spots.

Some simple steps can drastically reduce any risk from nail lamps.

How can I stop my nails from breaking?

Nails are subject to a lot of forces in everyday life. To withstand these without breaking, they need to be strong but still retain some flexibility.

Nail hydration tips
Water has a huge impact on nail properties. Too little water makes nails brittle so they crack instead of bending, but excess water makes them soft and weak.

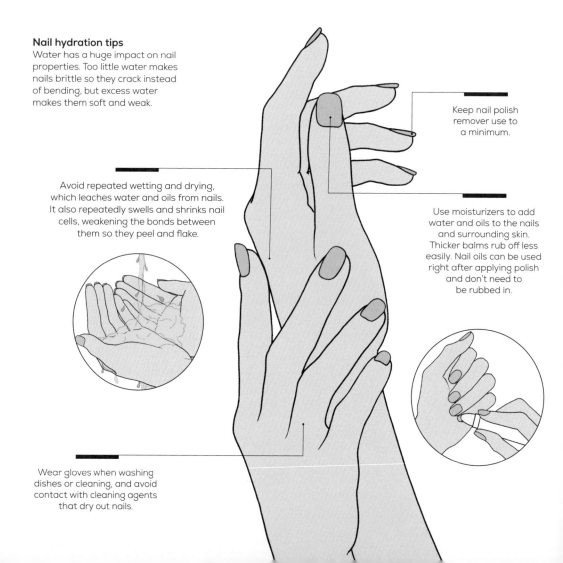

Keep nail polish remover use to a minimum.

Avoid repeated wetting and drying, which leaches water and oils from nails. It also repeatedly swells and shrinks nail cells, weakening the bonds between them so they peel and flake.

Use moisturizers to add water and oils to the nails and surrounding skin. Thicker balms rub off less easily. Nail oils can be used right after applying polish and don't need to be rubbed in.

Wear gloves when washing dishes or cleaning, and avoid contact with cleaning agents that dry out nails.

Nail strengtheners

Nail strengtheners can harden soft, bendy nails with ingredients that crosslink proteins. They can be used alone or as base coats.

For example, many strengtheners contain methylene glycol, a form of formaldehyde. Compared to hair treatments there's less product and no heat, so the risks are much lower. Use them in a well-ventilated area, and avoid skin contact. Overuse of formaldehyde strengtheners can make nails too inflexible, which can increase breakage.

Dimethyl urea and glyoxal work in a similar way, but penetrate less deeply into the nail so overuse is less of a problem. They are also less allergenic. Some nail strengthening products also contain similar ingredients to bond builders for hair, like maleic acid.

Other nail strengtheners contain nylon or silk fibres that add rigidity to the nail, or they may just be clear polishes that form a harder film.

> Adequate protein intake is needed for strong nails.

Nail supplements

Malnutrition can lead to weak nails, but there isn't strong evidence that supplements help much. Fingernails take six months to grow, so the impact of nutrition is generally quite delayed.

Since nails are made of protein, adequate protein intake is needed for strong nails. Weak nails can be a sign of biotin or iron deficiency. Some studies have found that 2.5mg of biotin a day may be able to improve very brittle nails. However, biotin can interfere with some blood tests.

A few studies suggest that silicon and collagen supplements may reduce breakage.

BEAUTY MYTHS

CALCIUM AND NAILS

Can calcium make nails stronger? Since calcium is only found in nails in trace amounts (0.1–0.2%), it's very unlikely that it would affect nail strength. A large study found no change in nail quality after a year of calcium supplementation.

NAIL STRENGTHENING

Methylene glycol releases formaldehyde which strengthens nails by crosslinking proteins, similar to hair treatments.

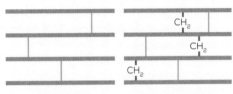

Natural nails
Crosslinking bonds join adjacent nail proteins to make a stronger structure.

With strengthener
Formaldehyde creates extra bonds between proteins to add strength and rigidity.

Why do my nails look different?

Changes in your nails can have many causes, from superficial damage and infections to serious underlying conditions like nutritional deficiencies, heart disease, or cancer.

A visual guide to nail changes
Here are some nail changes and their common causes. Any change without an obvious explanation should be checked out by a doctor.

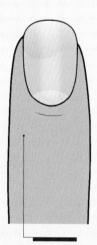

Yellow, orange, and green stains
Caused by nail polish pigments. These usually fade a few weeks after removing the polish, but deeper stains might need to grow out. Use a base coat to prevent these.

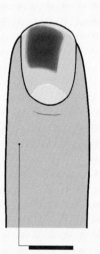

Green nails
Usually *Pseudomonas* bacterial infection, which can form under improperly applied or cracked artificial nails. This is best treated by a doctor, who may prescribe an antibiotic.

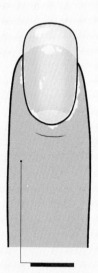

White powdery nails and skin
Often due to temporary dehydration with nail polish remover. Use removers with hydrating ingredients, or moisturize afterwards.

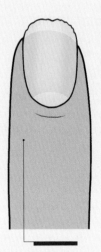

Brittle nails
Frequent nail breakage usually results from repeated exposure to water, or nutritional deficiencies (see p240).

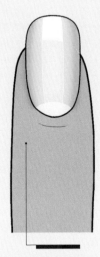

Yellow nails
Thickened, crumbly yellow nails usually indicate a fungal infection, which is best treated by a doctor.

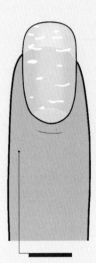

Nail pits or depressions
White spots and flakes are usually clumps of nail cells that have separated from the surface of the nail, such as with improper nail product removal.

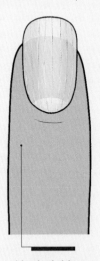

Vertical ridges
Ridges along the nail form when different parts of the nail matrix produce cells unevenly. This is more common with age.

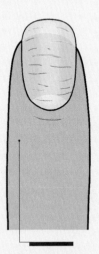

Horizontal ridges
Ridges across the nail usually come from trauma, such as picking at the nails. Very deep grooves can form during severe illness.

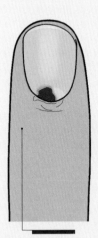

Dark marks
Injuries can cause a hemorrhage under the nail, which appears as a dark red or brown spot. Brown spots and streaks can also be melanomas.

Glossary

Active ingredients
Responsible for a product's main function. In skincare, these often produce a longer-lasting effect.

Alkali (alkaline)
Has a pH above 7. Also known as "basic".

Antioxidant
Substance that can neutralize reactive free radicals.

Bond
Chemical link between atoms.

Collagen
Protein that gives strength and support to connective tissues, including the skin's dermis.

Cortex
The inside of the hair, under the cuticle.

Crosslink
Bonds between separate chains that add strength and rigidity, like rungs on a ladder.

Cuticle
Thin outside layer of hair, or thin film of dead skin on the nail surface.

Dehydration
Removal of water.

Dermis
Middle layer of skin, under the epidermis, containing blood vessels, nerves, and hair follicles. Contributes to skin's strength, flexibility, and resilience.

Elastin
Protein that helps tissues return to their original shape after stretching. Found in the skin's dermis.

Emulsion
Mixture of liquids that normally don't mix together. Emulsions are named after the main liquids it contains e.g. an oil-in-water emulsion contains droplets of oil dispersed in water.

Endocrine disruptor
Substance that interferes with hormones to cause harmful health effects. Many common substances impact hormones to some extent, but most are not considered endocrine disruptors.

Enzyme
Type of protein that facilitates biological reactions, including essential metabolic processes inside our bodies.

Epidermis
Outermost layer of skin. Its main function is to create a barrier between us and our environment.

Exfoliation
Removal of dead cells from the skin's surface.

F-layer
Layer of lipids permanently bonded to the hair surface. Acts as a natural conditioner.

Free radicals
Highly reactive, unstable molecules. They are essential in biological function, but cause damage when they react with other parts of the body, especially when formed in excess. Their reactivity comes from unpaired electrons.

Hair follicle
Structure from which hair grows, containing the hair root.

Humectant
Ingredient that holds onto water. Often used for moisturizing.

Hydration
Addition of water.

Hydrogen bond
Type of bond, abundant in hair and nails, that contributes greatly to their strength and structure. Commonly formed by molecules that contain lots of nitrogen and oxygen, like proteins. Easily broken by water.

Hydrophilic
Attracted to water.

Hydrophobic
Repellent to water; usually also attracted to oil (lipophilic).

Hyperpigmentation
Excessive pigment production, resulting in darker patches of skin. Includes sun spots and post-acne marks.

Hypodermis
Deepest layer of skin, composed mostly of fat. Also called subcutaneous tissue.

Inflammation
Body's response to potential harm. Commonly involves redness and swelling.

Inorganic
Substances mostly based on elements aside from carbon.

Keratin
Tough protein found in skin, hair, and nails.

Lipids
Oily substances that don't dissolve in water. Often colloquially called "oils".

Melanin
Natural pigment that colours our skin and hair.

Melanoma
Uncommon but dangerous form of skin cancer, originating in melanocytes (melanin-producing cells).

Microbes
Microscopic organisms, such as bacteria, viruses, or fungi.

Occlusive
Ingredient that can act as a barrier to water. Often used for moisturizing.

Organic
In chemistry, this refers to substances based on the element carbon, often associated with living things.

Oxidation
Chemical process where electrons are lost, often involving oxygen or free radicals.

Oxidative stress
When there are too many free radicals for the body to neutralize, leading to increased damage. Thought to contribute to aging and many diseases.

pH
Measure of acidity or alkalinity. Water is neutral (pH 7). Acidic means the pH is below 7, while alkaline means the pH is above 7. An extreme pH in either direction can be corrosive. Our skin, hair, and nails are usually slightly acidic.

Polymer
Molecule containing many similar units joined into a long chain. Polymers include plastics, proteins, and starch.

Protein
Biological molecule made of many amino acids joined together.

Retinoids
Skincare ingredients that work like vitamin A, capable of addressing many common skin concerns.

Sebum
Oily mixture produced by sebaceous glands that lubricates the skin's surface. Often called "skin oil".

Skin turnover
Renewal of skin cells, as old cells are shed and new ones are produced.

Solvent
Substance that dissolves other substances. For example, water is a solvent for salt.

Stratum corneum
Outermost layer of epidermis containing dead skin cells. Often called the skin barrier.

Sun protection factor (SPF)
Measures how well a sunscreen protects against skin reddening and burning. Higher SPF means more protection.

Surfactant
Type of ingredient with a "head" that likes water, and a "tail" that likes oil. Classified by the charge of the head. Commonly used for cleaning, and stabilizing emulsions.

Toxicology
Study of the harmful effects of substances on living organisms.

Ultraviolet (UV)
Form of light that's more energetic than visible light, with shorter wavelengths. The most harmful part of sunlight.

Viscosity modifier
Ingredient used to thicken formulas.

Wavelength
Distance between two peaks in a wave, such as light. Light of different wavelengths have different colours. Shorter wavelengths are more energetic.

Bibliography

A full bibliography of sources referred to by the author as part of her research for this book can be found at:
www.dk.com/uk/information/science-of-beauty-biblio/

General references

Baki G, Alexander K. *Introduction to Cosmetic Formulation and Technology*, 1st ed; Wiley & Sons, 2015.

Baumann's Cosmetic Dermatology, 3rd ed; Baumann LS, Rieder EA, Sun MD, eds; McGraw Hill, 2022.

Cosmetic Dermatology: Products and Procedures, 3rd ed; Draelos ZD, ed; Wiley, 2022.

Robbins CR. *Chemical and Physical Behavior of Human Hair*; Springer, 2012.

Practical Modern Hair Science; Evans T, Wickett RR, eds; Allured Business Media, 2012.

Handbook of Cosmetic Science and Technology, 4th ed; Barel AO, Paye M, Maibach HI, eds; CRC Press, 2014.

Marsh J, Gray J, Tosti A. *Healthy Hair*, 1st ed; Springer, 2015.

Anastassakis A. *Androgenetic Alopecia From A to Z*, 1st ed; Springer Cham, 2022.

Principles and Practice of Photoprotection, 1st ed; Wang SQ, Lim HW, eds; Adis Cham, 2016.

Sunscreens: Regulations and Commercial Development, 3rd ed; Shaath N, ed; CRC Press, 2013.

Faulkner EB. *Coloring the Cosmetic World: Using Pigments in Decorative Cosmetic Formulations*, 2nd ed; John Wiley & Sons, 2021.

Morris R. *Makeup Masterclass*;

Rae Morris, 2016.

Schoon DD. *Nail Structure and Product Chemistry*, 2nd ed; Thomson Delmar Learning, 2005.

Textbook of Cosmetic Dermatology, 5th ed; Baran R, Maibach HI, eds; CRC Press, 2017.

Discovering Cosmetic Science; Barton S, Eastman A, Isom A, McLaverty D, Soong YL, eds; Royal Society of Chemistry, 2020.

Carli B. *Cosmetic Formulations: A Beginners Guide*, 7th ed; Institute of Personal Care Science, 2020.

What is beauty?

6 Trujillo LT, et al., *Cogn Affect Behav Neurosci*. 2014, doi:10.3758/s13415-013-0230-2 • Wong JS & Penner AM, *Res Soc Stratif Mobil*. 2016, doi:10.1016/j.rssm.2016.04.002 • Dove, *The Real Cost of Beauty Ideals*, 2022, deloitte.com/content/dam/assets-zone1/au/en/docs/services/economics/deloitte-au-economics-real-cost-beauty-ideals-041022.pdf

Beauty basics

18 Darbre PD, et al., *J Appl Toxicol*. 2004, doi:10.1002/jat.958 • Golden R, et al., *Crit Rev Toxicol*. 2005, doi:10.1080/10408440490920104 • Scientific Committee on Consumer Safety (SCCS), Opinion on Propylparaben, 2021, health.ec.europa.eu/system/files/2022-08/sccs_o_243.pdf • European Commission, Consumers: Commission improves safety of cosmetics, 2014, ec.europa.eu/commission/presscorner/detail/en/IP_14_1051 • Fransway AF, et al., *Dermatitis* 2019, doi:10.1097/

DER.0000000000000429 • International Fragrance Association, Introduction: The IFRA Standards, ifrafragrance.org/safe-use/introduction • Scientific Committee on Consumer Products (SCCP), Opinion on Phthalates in Cosmetic Products, 2007, ec.europa.eu/health/ph_risk/committees/04_sccp/docs/sccp_o_106.pdf

30 Churchill A, et al., *Food Qual Prefer*. 2009, doi:10.1016/j.foodqual.2009.02.002

37 Gonçalves GMS, et al., *Braz Arch Biol Technol*. 2013, doi:10.1590/S1516-89132013000200005

42 National Research Council, Review of Fate, Exposure, and Effects of Sunscreens in Aquatic Environments and Implications for Sunscreen Usage and Human Health, The National Academies Press, 2022, nap.nationalacademies.org/catalog/26381/review-of-fate-exposure-and-effects-of-sunscreens-in-aquatic-environments-and-implications-for-sunscreen-usage-and-human-health • Sudhakar U, This Indian tree prized by Chinese royalty is on the road to extinction, *The Times of India*, 2022, m.timesofindia.com/india/this-indian-tree-prized-by-chinese-royalty-is-on-the-road-to-extinction/amp_articleshow/88967537.cms • Gemedzhieva N, et al., *Sweet dreams: Assessing opportunities and threats in Kazakhstan's wild liquorice root trade*, TRAFFIC, 2021, traffic.org/publications/reports/a-sweet-tooth-for-medicinal-liquorice-a-risk-to-ecosystems-and-livelihoods-warns-a-new-report-released-this-world-health-day • Golsteijn L, et al.,

Integr Environ Assess Manag. 2018, doi:10.1002/ieam.4064 • Kröhnert H & Stucki M, *Sustainability* 2021, doi:10.3390/su13158478 • Herbes C, et al., *J Clean Prod.* 2018, doi:10.1016/j.jclepro.2018.05.106

46 European Commission, Directorate-General for Environment, *Second Report from the Commission to the Council and the European Parliament on the statistics on the number of animals used for experimental and other scientific purposes in the Member States of the European Union*, Publications Office, 1999, op.europa.eu/en/publication-detail/-/publication/bdd270d6-3cbd-494b-a1bd-fe64ed6ed52a • The Humane Society of the United States, Timeline: Cosmetics testing on animals, 2023, humanesociety.org/resources/timeline-cosmetics-testing-animals • Bjerke DL, et al., Skin sensitization next generation risk assessment framework and case study, 2022, cir-safety.org/sites/default/files/160th%20CIR%20EP%20Skin%20Sensitization%20NAM%20Upate%20Don%20Bjerke%20Final%20updated.pdf

50 Dermnet, Skin changes in pregnancy, 2021, dermnetnz.org/topics/skin-changes-in-pregnancy • MotherSafe: NSW Medications in Pregnancy and Breastfeeding Service, Skin Care, Hair Care and Cosmetic Treatments in Pregnancy and Breastfeeding, 2021, seslhd.health.nsw.gov.au/sites/default/files/groups/Royal_Hospital_for_Women/Mothersafe/documents/skinhaircareandcosmetictreatments april2021.pdf

Everyday skincare

57 Czarnowicki T, et al., *J Allergy Clin Immunol.* 2016, doi:10.1016/j.jaci.2015.08.013 • Man MQ &

Elias PM, *Clin Interv Aging.* 2019, doi:10.2147/cia.s235595 • Wen S, et al., *J Eur Acad Dermatol Venereol.* 2022, doi:10.1111/jdv.18360

59 Abbas S, et al., *Dermatol Ther.* 2004, doi:10.1111/j.1396-0296.2004.04s1004.x • Korting HC & Braun-Falco O, *Clin Dermatol.* 1996, doi:10.1016/0738-081x(95)00104-n

64 Sendrasoa FA, et al., *Allergy Asthma Clin Immunol.* 2020, doi:10.1186/s13223-019-0398-2 • Kong F, et al., *Arch Derm Res.* 2017, doi:10.1007/s00403-017-1764-x • Vashi NA, et al., *J Clin Aesthet Dermatol.* 2016, PMID:26962390.

67 Raghunath RS, et al., *Clin Exp Dermatol.* 2015, doi:10.1111/ced.12588

71 Oyetakin-White P, et al., *Clin Exp Dermatol.* 2015, doi:10.1111/ced.12455 • Axelsson J, et al., *BMJ.* 2010, doi:10.1136/bmj.c6614

74 Baldwin H & Tan J, *Am J Clin Dermatol.* 2021, doi:10.1007/s40257-020-00542-y • Fam VW, et al., *Nutrients.* 2020, doi:10.3390/nu12113581

77 Mac-Mary S, et al., *Skin Res Technol.* 2006, doi:10.1111/j.0909-752x.2006.00160.x • Palma ML, et al., *Skin Res Technol.* 2015, doi:10.1111/srt.12208 • Rodrigues L, et al., *Clin Cosmet Investig Dermatol.* 2015, doi:10.2147/ccid.s86822

80 Lupi O, et al., *J Cosmet Dermatol.* 2007, doi:10.1111/j.1473-2165.2007.00304.x • Gye J, et al., *Australas J Dermatol.* 2014, doi:10.1111/ajd.12133 • Marcos LA & Kahler R, *Int J Infect Dis.* 2015, doi:10.1016/j.ijid.2015.07.004

84 Australian Skin and Skin Cancer Research Centre, Position statement: Balancing the harms

and benefits of sun exposure, 2023, assc.org.au/wp-content/uploads/2023/01/Sun-Exposure-Summit-PositionStatement_V1.9.pdf

86 Lopes FCPS, et al., *JAMA Dermatol.* 2021, doi:10.1001/jamadermatol.2020.4616 • Coelho SG, et al., *Pigment Cell Melanoma Res.* 2015, doi:10.1111/pcmr.12331 • Rawlings AV, *Int J Cosmet Sci.* 2006, doi:10.1111/j.1467-2494.2006.00302.x • Brenner M & Hearing VJ, *Photochem Photobiol.* 2008, doi:10.1111/j.1751-1097.2007.00226.x • Fajuyigbe D & Young AR, *Pigment Cell Melanoma Res.* 2016, doi:10.1111/pcmr.12511 • Faurschou A & Wulf HC, *Photodermatol Photoimmunol Photomed.* 2004, doi:10.1111/j.1600-0781.2004.00118.x • The International Agency for Research on Cancer Working Group on artificial ultraviolet (UV) light and skin cancer, *Int J Cancer.* 2007, doi:10.1002/ijc.22453 • Holman DM, et al., *JAMA Dermatol.* 2018, doi:10.1001/jamadermatol.2018.0028

89 Cole C, et al., *Photodermatol Photoimmunol Photomed.* 2016, doi:10.1111/phpp.12214

90 International Organization for Standardization, *In vivo determination of the sun protection factor (SPF)* (ISO 24444:2019), International Organization for Standardization, 2019, iso.org/standard/72250.html • International Organization for Standardization, *Determination of sunscreen UVA photoprotection in vitro* (ISO 24443:2021), International Organization for Standardization, 2022, iso.org/standard/75059.html • Reinau D, et al., *Br J Dermatol.* 2015, doi:10.1111/bjd.14015 • Zundell MP, et al., *JEADV Clinical Practice.* 2023, doi:10.1002/jvc2.251 • Petersen

B & Wulf HC, *Photodermatol Photoimmunol Photomed*. 2014, doi:10.1111/phpp.12099 • Schneider J, *Arch Dermatol*. 2002, doi:10.1001/archderm.138.6.838-b

92 Toxicology Section, Scientific Evaluation Branch, *Literature review on the safety of titanium dioxide and zinc oxide nanoparticles in sunscreens*, Therapeutic Goods Administration, 2016, tga.gov.au/resources/publication/publications/literature-review-safety-titanium-dioxide-and-zinc-oxide-nanoparticles-sunscreens • Iannacone MR, et al., *Photodermatol Photoimmunol Photomed*. 2014, doi:10.1111/phpp.12109

94 Gambichler T, et al., *BMC Dermatol*. 2001, doi:10.1186/1471-5945-1-6 • Wong JCF, et al., *Photodermatol Photoimmunol Photomed*. 1996, doi:10.1111/j.1600-0781.1996.tb00189.x • Utrillas MP, et al., *Photochem Photobiol*. 2010, doi:10.1111/j.1751-1097.2009.00677.x • Turner J & Parisi A, *Int J Environ Res Public Health*. 2018, doi:10.3390/ijerph15071507 • Sebaratnam D, Vitamin B3, niacinamide and reducing skin cancer risk: what does the research say?, The Conversation, 2022, theconversation.com/vitamin-b3-niacinamide-and-reducing-skin-cancer-risk-what-does-the-research-say-177729 • Jesus A, et al., *Antioxidants (Basel)*. 2023, doi:10.3390/antiox12010138

Skincare specifics

108 Xin C, et al., *J Cosmet Dermatol*. 2021, doi:10.1111/jocd.13452 • Branchet MC, et al., *Gerontology* 1990, doi:10.1159/000213172 • Reilly DM & Lozano J, *Plast Aesthet Res*. 2021, doi:10.

20517/2347-9264.2020.153 • Lephart ED, *Ageing Res Rev*. 2016, doi:10.1016/j.arr.2016.08.001

114 Friedmann D, et al., *Clin Cosmet Investig Dermatol*. 2017, doi:10.2147/ccid.s95830

118 Gómez DM, et al., *Tren Med*. 2019, doi:10.15761/tim.1000210 • Mills OH Jr, et al., *Int J Dermatol*. 1986, doi:10.1111/j.1365-4362.1986.tb04534.x

136 Conti A, et al., *Int J Cosmet Sci*. 1996, doi:10.1111/j.1467-2494.1996.tb00131.x

Hair

168 Lee Y, et al., *Ann Dermatol*. 2011, doi:10.5021/ad.2011.23.4.455

Makeup

184 Monnot AD, et al., *Food Chem Toxicol*. 2015, doi:10.1016/j.fct.2015.03.022

187 Gelest, Microparticle Surface Modification: Innovating Particle Functionalization, 2009, technical. gelest.com/brochures/microparticle-surface-modification/innovating-particle-functionalization

200 Petersen B & Wulf HC, *Photodermatol Photoimmunol Photomed*. 2014, doi:10.1111/phpp.12099 • Scientific Committee on Consumer Safety, SCCS Notes of Guidance for the Testing of Cosmetic Ingredients and their Safety Evaluation 11th revision, 2021, health.ec.europa.eu/publications/sccs-notes-guidance-testing-cosmetic-ingredients-and-their-safety-evaluation-11th-revision_en

210 Ciolino JB, et al., *Ophthal*

Plast Reconstr Surg. 2009, doi:10.1097/iop.0b013e3181ab443e • Pack LD, et al., *Optometry* 2008, doi:10.1016/j.optm.2008.02.011

212 The Cosmetic, Toiletry and Perfumery Association, PFAS and cosmetics – the facts, thefactsabout.co.uk/news/pfas-and-cosmetics-andndash-the-facts • US Food & Drug Administration, Talc, 2022, fda.gov/cosmetics/cosmetic-ingredients/talc • O'Brien KM, et al., *JAMA*. 2020, doi:10.1001/jama.2019.20079

216 Matsushita S, et al., *J Cosmet Sci*. 2015, PMID:26454904

Nails

220 Wang B, et al., *Prog Mater Sci*. 2016, doi:10.1016/j.pmatsci.2015.06.001 • Baswan S, et al., *Mycoses*. 2017, doi:10.1111/myc.12592 • Walters KA & Lane ME in *Cosmetic Formulation: Principles and Practice*; Benson HAE, Roberts MS, Leite-Silva VR & Walters K, eds; CRC Press, 2019.

226 Mendelsohn E, et al., *Environ Int*. 2016, doi:10.1016/j.envint.2015.10.005

236 Lamplugh A, et al., *Environ Pollut*. 2019, doi:10.1016/j.envpol.2019.03.086

239 Baeza D, et al., *Photochem Photobiol Sci*. 2018, doi:10.1039/c7pp00388a

240 Lipner S, *J Drugs Dermatol*. 2020, doi:10.36849/jdd.2020.4946

Image credits

The publisher would like to thank the following for their kind permission to reproduce their photographs:

(Key: a-above; b-below/bottom; c-centre; f-far; l-left; r-right; t-top)

7 Getty Images / iStock: Sasha Brazhnik. **32-33 Getty Images / iStock:** Svetlana Borisova. **34-35 Getty Im** Moment / Iryna Veklich. **40-41 Dreamstime.com:** Anakimfor. **43 Dreamstime.com:** Anastasiia Bidzilia (bl). **Getty Images:** fStop / Norman Posselt (bc); Moment / Elena Noviello (br). **60-61 Getty Images / iStock:** gilas. **76-77 Getty Images:** Moment / Maryna Terletska (bc). **122-123 Getty Images / iStock:** Ekaterina Klishevnik.
131 Getty Images / iStock: Ekaterina Klishevnik. **162-163 Getty Images / iStock:** Ekaterina Klishevnik. **180 Getty Images:** Moment / mikroman6 (bl, bc/Red, br, bc). **181 Dreamstime.com:** Viktoriya89 (tr). **Getty Images:** Moment / mikroman6 (bc, br). **Shutterstock.com:** Meowcyber (bl). **186 Depositphotos Inc:** artcasta. **193 Dreamstime.com:** Dmitryi Epov (crb/Brush.9); Sharlotta Ulrikh (cra/x3, crb/Brush.7). **Shutterstock. com:** Foonia (tr, cr, br); Pixel-Shot (cra, crb). **196 Dreamstime.com:** Anstasiya Malysheva (tr). **Getty Images / iStock:** moonHo Joe (ca). **197 Dreamstime. com:** Chernetskaya (tl); Tatyanaego (tl/Eyeliner pen); Anstasiya Malysheva (tc); Kozpho (cra). **209 Getty Images / iStock:** Svetlana Borisova. **210-211 Getty Images / iStock:** bonetta (b). **211 Dreamstime.com:** L M (br). **Getty Images / iStock:** imagehub88 (cra). **212-213 Getty Images / iStock:** Floortje. **222 Dreamstime.com:** Sergey Kolesnikov (bl). **225 Getty Images / iStock:** Beeldbewerking (bl). **226-227 Getty Images:** Westend61 (t)

All other images © Dorling Kindersley

Index

Author's acknowledgments

This book would not be possible without the combined efforts of many people. I am forever indebted to:

The experts whose feedback improved this book immensely: Esther Olu, Dr Annika Lagut, Dr Amber O Evans, Larry Yeo, Ruby Golani, Dr Anke Ginzburg, Dr Mara Evangelista-Huber, Stephen Ko, and Ruby.

My colleagues whose knowledge and advice informed much of this book. Special thanks go to Jen Novakovich, Dr Frédéric Lebreux, Belinda Carli, TRI Princeton, Dr Anjali Mahto, Hannah English, Lalita Iyer, and Dr Davin Lim, as well as the scientists and educators listed in the bibliography.

The DK team who brought this project to life, patiently wrangling my ideas into a book far better than I thought possible: Amy Slack, Sarah Snelling, Emma Hill, and Emma and Tom Forge.

The sponsors whose financial assistance has allowed me to make science communication my career. I am extremely grateful that you see the value in my work.

The mentors and colleagues who honed my science and communication skills, especially my former students, my PhD supervisor Prof Kate Jolliffe, and my colleagues at Matrix Education, in particular DJ Kim, Dr Alex Argyros, Vivian Law, and Louise Donnelly. Thanks also to Christina Butcher, the Gushcloud team and the Vengadoras for their invaluable business-related guidance.

My friends and family, especially my incredible partner Omar, whose generous emotional and practical support allows my work (and me) to exist.

Most importantly: you, my readers and followers, for supporting me and seeking science, even though it takes increasing effort to see past misinformation. Thank you for always being a source of inspiration.

Publisher's acknowledgments

DK would like to thank Sibel Ekemen, Vicky Read, and Josef Mayfield for early design work on the book, Nigel Wright (XAB Design) for photographic styling, Usman Ansari for image retouching, Katie Hewitt for proofreading, and Vanessa Bird for indexing.

About the Author

Dr Michelle Wong is the science communicator and chemist behind Lab Muffin Beauty Science, where she explains the science behind beauty, and helps consumers make better decisions about their products. Founded in 2011, Lab Muffin Beauty Science now has over a million followers across Instagram, YouTube, and TikTok. She also works as a product development and science communication consultant.

Through her science communication work, Michelle has partnered with many well-known brands including L'Oréal and P&G, and delivered an invited talk at Google News Initiative's APAC Trusted Media Summit. Her work has been featured in publications including *Wired*, *The New York Times*, *Elle*, *The Atlantic*, *Chemistry & Engineering News*, and *Cosmetics & Toiletries*. She has co-hosted several online cosmetic science conferences, and is the co-founder of Beauty SciComm, an initiative to boost the quality, volume and reach of accurate beauty science content. She has an eBook, The Lab Muffin Guide to Basic Skincare, and cohosted Adore Beauty's Skincare School podcast.

She holds a bachelor of advanced science (first class honours with university medal), a PhD in chemistry (medicinal and supramolecular chemistry), and a diploma of cosmetic formulation.

You can find Michelle online at:
YouTube: @LabMuffinBeautyScience
Instagram: @labmuffinbeautyscience
TikTok: @labmuffinbeautyscience
Website: labmuffin.com

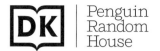

DK LONDON
Senior Acquisitions Editors Zara Anvari, Becky Alexander
Managing Editor Clare Double
Acquisitions Editor Amy Slack
Senior Designer Sarah Snelling
Senior Production Editor Tony Phipps
Production Controller Stephanie McConnell
Jacket Designer Sarah Snelling
Jacket and Sales Material Co-ordinator Emily Cannings
Art Director Maxine Pedliham
Publishing Director Katie Cowan

Editorial Emma Hill
Design Emma Forge, Tom Forge
Illustration Montana Forbes
Photography Sun Lee

First published in Great Britain in 2024 by
Dorling Kindersley Limited
DK, One Embassy Gardens, 8 Viaduct Gardens,
London, SW11 7BW

The authorised representative in the EEA is
Dorling Kindersley Verlag GmbH. Arnulfstr. 124,
80636 Munich, Germany

10 9 8 7 6 5 4 3 2 1
001–339261–Jun/2024

A CIP catalogue record for this book
is available from the British Library.
ISBN: 978-0-2416-5699-0

Printed and bound in China

www.dk.com

This book was made with Forest
Stewardship Council™ certified
paper – one small step in DK's
commitment to a sustainable future.
Learn more at **www.dk.com/uk/
information/sustainability**